T0130626

STUCK

STUCK

How Vaccine Rumors Start—and Why They
Don't Go Away

Heidi J. Larson, PhD

PROFESSOR

DEPARTMENT OF INFECTIOUS DISEASE EPIDEMIOLOGY

LONDON SCHOOL OF HYGIENE & TROPICAL MEDICINE

LONDON, UK

AND

DEPARTMENT OF HEALTH METRICS SCIENCES

UNIVERSITY OF WASHINGTON

SEATTLE, USA

OXFORD
UNIVERSITY PRESS

OXFORD
UNIVERSITY PRESS

Oxford University Press is a department of the University of Oxford. It furthers
the University's objective of excellence in research, scholarship, and education
by publishing worldwide. Oxford is a registered trade mark of Oxford University
Press in the UK and certain other countries.

Published in the United States of America by Oxford University Press
198 Madison Avenue, New York, NY 10016, United States of America.

Library of Congress Cataloging-in-Publication Data
Name: Larson, J. Heidi, author.
Title: Stuck : how vaccine rumors start—and why they don't go away /
[Heidi J. Larson].
Description: New York, NY : Oxford University Press, [2020] |
Includes bibliographical references and index.
Identifiers: LCCN 2020005847 (print) | LCCN 2020005848 (ebook) |
ISBN 9780190077242 (hardback) | ISBN 9780190077259 (epub)
Subjects: LCSH: Vaccination—Public opinion. | Immunization—
Public opinion. | Anti-vaccination movement. | Communication in public health. |
Public health—Citizen participation. | Rumor.
Classification: LCC RA638 .L37 2020 (print) | LCC RA638 (ebook) |
DDC 614.4/7—dc23
LC record available at https://lccn.loc.gov/2020005847
LC ebook record available at https://lccn.loc.gov/2020005848

5 7 9 8 6
Printed by Sheridan Books, Inc., United States of America

The present epoch is one of these critical moments in which the thought of mankind is undergoing a process of transformation.

Two fundamental factors are at the base of this transformation. The first is the destruction of those religious, political, and social beliefs in which all the elements of our civilisation are rooted. The second is the creation of entirely new conditions of existence and thought as the result of modern scientific and industrial discoveries.

The ideas of the past, although half destroyed, being still very powerful, and the ideas which are to replace them being still in process of formation, the modern age represents a period of transition and anarchy.

—Gustave Le Bon, *The Crowd: A Study of the Popular Mind* (1896)

CONTENTS

ACKNOWLEDGMENTS

The concept and research for this book has been a journey evolving over the past decade, with most of the writing in the past few years, while the turbulence around this topic intensified.

My views have not always been welcomed, as they question some of modus operandi of the public health community and give voice to some of the uncomfortable concerns and questions expressed by the public that I feel we, as a scientific and public health community, need to hear. We can sit in our bubble of mutual recognition of the value of vaccines, with our achievements defined by the number of people vaccinated, but that model is quickly becoming outdated. The challenges are far deeper as explored in *Stuck*.

My source of strength—not only for the writing of this book, but for standing up for what I believe—has been Peter. From singing "Don't let the bastards grind you down" to cooking the most spectacular meals and cheering me on while I used precious summer holidays, nights, and weekends to write this book, I don't know how I would have soldiered through to get this book finished without his unending patience, love, and support.

Although my parents are no longer alive, my father in particular would have smiled seeing the activist spirit alive and well. My stepmother Pat and family, brother Jeffrey and family, stepchildren, and grandchildren have all been a joy and support throughout.

At the Press, Chad Zimmerman was a tremendous help as I navigated and responded to the multiple reviews of the initial book proposal and outline, always asking me the right questions and giving me thoughtful feedback throughout the writing process. Sarah Humphreville and the Oxford University Press team who handled the last leg of the impressively choreographed production-to-marketing journey have been a pleasure to work with.

In terms of the research that built the foundation for this book, I particularly want to thank Walt Orenstein and Michael Galway who, just over a decade ago in their roles at the Bill & Melinda Gates Foundation, understood the need for this research and went against the mainstream to help us get our first grant to establish in 2010 what has become The Vaccine Confidence Project™.

Thanks to that grant, I was able to hire Pauline Paterson and Lee Barker to help get our research started and build our media monitoring system and database. I also want to thank our first collaborators Larry Madoff and John Brownstein who helped us transform a media monitoring platform to detect disease outbreaks to a platform to detect vaccine rumors and misinformation that we assessed as possibly posing risks to immunization programs.

Another invaluable part of the grant was the support to convene an International Advisory Board who brought crucial insights and asked us important questions to consider as we built the longer-term strategy for the Project. I want to thank all the IAC members, many of whom continued to stay engaged with our work: Roy Anderson, Narendra Kumar Arora, Madhava Ram Balakrishnan, Jan Bonhoeffer, Louis Cooper, Ciro de Quadros, Michael Galway,

Robert Goble, Adenike Grange, Kenneth Hartigan-Go, David Heymann, Samuel Katz, Najwa Khuri-bulos, Raj Kumar, Julie Leask, Glen Nowak, and Patrick Zuber.

Others who lent their valuable insights in the early stages of the Vaccine Confidence Project were Zulfiqar Bhutta, Leszek Borysiewicz, Gabrielle Fitzgerald, Adel Mahmoud, Ed Marcuse, Paul Offit, Saad Omer, Muhammad Pate, Stanley Plotkin, and Helen Reese. I am also grateful for being invited to chair a novel round-table organized by Angus Thompson and Michael Watson in 2010, as the discussions across the diverse participants raised important questions for our research and unearthed some stories reflected on in the book.

I want to acknowledge the WHO Strategic Advisory Group of Experts (SAGE) Working Group on Vaccine Hesitancy, which I participated in, as it was a significant forum established in 2012 to map the determinants of vaccine hesitancy and recommend strategies to address what was finally becoming recognized as a growing problem. Some of the issues raised in *Stuck* were influenced by our discussions in the Working Group. Other members in the group included: Mohuya Chaudhuri, Eve Dubé, Philippe Duclos, Juhani Eskola, Bruce Gellin, Susan Goldstein, Mahamane Laouali, Xiaofeng Liang, Noni MacDonald, Arthur Reingold, Melanie Schuster, Dilian Francisca Toro Torres, Kinzang Tshering, and Yuqing Zhou.

Finally, I particularly want to acknowledge and thank all those who have worked with me in building the Vaccine Confidence Project and who have been a constant inspiration. We have together created a tremendous global resource of case studies, new research methods, and a global mapping of vaccine emotions and beliefs over time and place which I refer to in a number of chapters in the book. The researchers include: Muhammed Afolabi, Abrar Alasmari,

Rachel Alter, Daniel Artus, Lee Barker, Eric Berger, Christy Braham, Tracey Chantler, Ai Ling Chiam, Jeremy Chiu, Richard Clarke, Sara Dada, Julia Darko, Roshan Daryanani, Daniel Epstein, Alexandre de Figueiredo, Kristen de Graaf, Chermain Denny, Jay Dowle, Robyn Eakle, Elisabeth Eckersberger, Luisa Enria, Michelle Fong, Mark Francis, Isaac Ghinai, Sophie Gregg, Kaiyi Han, Valerie Heywood, Suzanne Hurst, Caitlin Jarret, Emilie Karafillakis, Eliz Kilich, Antonis Kousoulis, Per Kummerwold, Shelley Lees, Zachary Levine Tatjana Marks, Sam Martin, Sandra Mounier-Jack, Gillian McKay, Thomas Mooney, Astrid Parys, Pauline Paterson, Dorothy Peprah, Simon Piatek, Eleanor Reynolds, Rachel Pool, Mahesh Rawal, William Schulz, Michiyo Shima, Clarissa Simas, David MD Smith, Elisabeth Smout, Fiona Sun, Neisha Sundaram, Angus Tengbeh, Daria Tserkovnay, Emily Warren, Katie Whitehurst, and Rose Wilson. While we have a growing global network of collaborators, I want to acknowledge some of our longer-term colleagues who have influenced my thinking as I wrote *Stuck*: Sumeet Agarwal, Nick Jones, Robert Kanwagi, Nduku Kilonzo, Gabriel Leung, Chris Murray, Robert Peckham, Lance Rodewald, James Rubin, Pierre VanDamme, Alex Vorsters, Mitchell Weiss, Charles Wiysonge, and Joe Wu. I also want to thank Johnny Heald, Ijaz and Sara Gilani for their enthusiastic support and ongoing collaboration in running our Vaccine Confidence Index™ since 2015, which has generated some of the insights referred to in *Stuck*.

There are many individuals whose thoughts, questions, and perspectives have helped shape the themes and writing of *Stuck*. Thank you. This is a time where the world is seeking a "new normal." Many of the conversations I had around *Stuck* were about the need for a new normal, before COVID-19 struck. Now we have no excuse. There is no "normal" to inhibit our new thinking.

PROLOGUE

On January 28, 2020, the final manuscript for this book moved from the editorial desks of the Press into production. Two days later, the World Health Organization (WHO) declared that a novel coronavirus outbreak, which started quietly in Wuhan, China, had become a "Public Health Emergency of International Concern." At the time of the January 30 WHO announcement, there were over 7,000 cases confirmed, 12,000 cases suspected, and 170 deaths in China, and the now named "COVID-19" virus had spread to 18 countries.

By early May 2020, the virus had spread to every region of the world, infecting over 3.5 million people and killing nearly 250,000. And, for some parts of the world, this was just the beginning.

In many ways, I am glad to have been able to finish this book before the COVID-19 pandemic shook the world—at every level. If my last months of writing would have been engulfed by the coronavirus context, it would have been difficult to not bring the experience of the pandemic into every chapter of this book in the same way that it has permeated and significantly altered personal and societal lives, politics, the economy, livelihoods, schooling, sports, and—in an ironic positive twist—climate change debates, as it gave the world a glimpse of what it takes to clear the skies of pollution with the near-halt of global air travel.

But, had that happened, it would have changed what *Stuck* is meant to be about, which is the myriad of (pre-COVID-19) societal, technological, and political influences that have changed the public's relationship with vaccines and what they stand for. It is about an era where vaccines, on the one hand, gained public acceptance to become as normal as brushing your teeth to one where every last ingredient in a vaccine is being questioned and debated.

Although this book is largely focused on the evolving dynamics around vaccines and the ferment which lies beneath, as I reread through the chapters while living in lockdown in London and watching countries around the world manage their pandemic responses differently, it struck me that the themes in *Stuck* are each highly relevant to how we manage and recover from this "emergency of international concern" and build a new future.

The first chapter is about rumors, reflecting on rumors as a kind of collective problem solving and a means to manage uncertainty through sharing evolving pieces of yet unverified information and gathering the views of others. Rumors thrive in situations of uncertainty whether around a new vaccine, unfamiliar disease outbreak or more catastrophic events like wars, natural disasters, or pandemics. While hostile and purposefully disruptive rumors and disinformation have been at the forefront of media attention, rumors can carry important pieces of new information, especially as a new situation unfolds like the novel coronavirus pandemic. Managing the fine line between intentionally harmful rumors and uncertain yet potentially invaluable ones is particularly fraught in authoritarian states eager to control the narrative, particularly in time of emergencies. We have seen a range of leaders, from those who tout unverified information about bleach cures to those repressing crucial information on the virus spread. In China, Dr. Li Wenliang sounded a clarion call through his social media posts, warning of a dangerous virus emerging in the Wuhan hospital where he worked, but was then confronted by state officials and forced to sign a statement that his message was an illegal rumor. Repressing information has been rife in a number of countries where leaders try to calm publics and send a signal "Keep Calm and Carry On" or "all under control" when publics know better.

A key theme throughout the book is the persistence of rumors—what sparks them, how they spread like a contagious virus, and how they hibernate until they find new fertile ground to re-emerge. Rumors around possible "cleansing" treatments and conspiracies that 5G technology causes COVID-19 are not new in the context of coronavirus but are older rumors which found a new opportunity to thrive. In 2003, the new 3G technology was suspected to cause SARS and, in 2009, new rumors circulated that the upgraded 4G technology caused Swine flu. Despite the various pronouncements by national and international agencies that viruses cannot travel on radio waves and mobile networks, rumors persist. Similarly, bleach cures have been (dangerously) advocated as a cure for autism, cancers, and now coronavirus.

Dignity and distrust and the sense of having no voice, feeling controlled by elites who are insensitive to the felt needs and concerns of the public, is another theme in the book—and a driver of vaccine dissent—which resonates with some of the public's experience of feeling controlled by the state during the pandemic response. Others feel left out when given instructions to "work at home," seemingly ignoring large sectors of the population whose work is not transportable. Dignity has also taken a toll in other ways with racist sentiment, stigmatization, and even physical aggression toward diaspora

Chinese and East Asian communities around the world, but also is at play within Chinese speaking communities with particular negativity expressed toward those from mainland China where the virus was first identified. While some of the sentiments are born out of anxiety and fear of catching the virus, and not uncommon in new and unknown disease outbreaks, the risk of contagion in some cases becomes an excuse to unearth and express already brewing "anti-other" sentiments and grievances. These experiences will live long in individual and collective memories, and risk undermining public trust and needed social cooperation around a new COVID-19 vaccine or other measures in the journey to "return to normal."

Chapter 3 is on risk, which is all about making decisions in the context uncertainty and chance. While *Stuck* is primarily about the many layers of influences on vaccine decisions, the COVID-19 pandemic has been a time of acute uncertainty and risks, with no vaccine yet available and the only prevention options being isolation, distancing, and hand washing. Scientific understanding has been evolving, with new learnings every day since the late December 2019 news of a not-yet-named new virus. Guidance for clinicians as well as the public has also been learning-while-doing, sometimes sending confusing messages to already anxious populations around the world. As with many crises, whether man-made or natural disasters, multiple risks often converge. In addition to the tremendous toll on health and lives lost due to the virus itself, the global economic crisis which has ensued has created other survival risks. At the end of the day, in the COVID-19 context, politicians as well as citizens need to weigh multiple risks as they make decisions. Some may accept a COVID-19 vaccine not because of its relative health benefit over any risks it may bear, but because it allows them to go back to work.

The volatility of opinion and protests around freedom of choice and voice is another thread throughout the book, which resonates deeply in the context of government-directed COVID-19 related lockdowns, isolation, and social distancing. The libertarian sentiments which drove the early demonstrations against compulsory smallpox vaccination in the 1800s to contemporary revolts against vaccine mandates are similar, in part, to the emotions which fueled protests against lockdown in multiple US cities, but in other parts of the world such as in India, the angry protests were partly a cry for survival as lockdowns cut the lifeline for migrant workers and hunger became a bigger issue than disease. In other countries, previous protests for social change and freedoms became wrapped into revolts against government COVID-19 restrictions. Like the stories in *Stuck*, where vaccine resistance is portrayed as being driven by deeper grievances, government controls in the name of COVID-19 can unearth deep-rooted angers against the state. As one *WIRED* article aptly titled "The Anti-Quarantine Protests Aren't About Covid-19" concluded, issues from gun rights to immigration, medical freedoms and abortion were the real roots of dissent.

Emotional contagion and the power of belief are other themes in *Stuck*, particularly as they relate to publics with anxieties around vaccines and those seeking more "natural" alternatives to build their immune system. In the context of COVID-19, publics reacted with panic buying—from masks and hand sanitizers to toilet paper and food staples. Alternative cures and prevention potions have flourished in the absence of an available proven treatment or vaccine—from the herbal "COVID Organic" cure, bottled and distributed in some African countries, to eating garlic and taking supplements promoted by homeopaths claiming they build your immune system to protect against catching the new coronavirus.

The last chapter of this book—On Pandemics and Publics— reflects on the experience of previous pandemics and calls out the urgency to better prepare for the next big one.

> *The world was lucky that the anticipated fatalities of the 2009 H1N1 pandemic were far less than expected. But if the world responds to the next high-risk pandemic with the same level of vaccine reluctance it did in response to H1N1, we may not be so lucky. It is time to not only understand what went wrong, but to start acting on it to build the public's trust—and the public health community's trustworthiness— before the next pandemic hits.*

The next pandemic has now hit. We do not have a vaccine (yet), but in the absence of a vaccine there is time to prepare, to build needed trust. Public compliance with social distancing and isolation and managing the economic and psychological costs of closing workplaces, schools, and travel, have tested our ability to cooperate. It has been a time of anxiety, creativity, caring, patience, impatience, fears, and hopes. How this plays out on willingness to accept a COVID-19 vaccine is unclear. It depends on where you live, how your community and country have treated you during this crisis, who you feel you can trust, whether you were close enough to someone whose life was nearly taken by the virus to know the real risks, and whether we have an available vaccine while the threat of the disease is still looming.

We are yet to see how we will emerge from this crisis. Perhaps we have been shaken enough to get unstuck from our old ways and be open to a new future.

Perhaps.

HJL

May 12, 2020

INTRODUCTION

It was winter in India. I was sitting in a holy cow and Krishna-adorned taxi in New Delhi, driving to meet colleagues working in the Ministry of Health. We were stuck in traffic, with a cacophony of impatient horns sounding in the background. The polluted smog was thick, so taking a deep breath to stay calm was not an option. I looked out the window—a movie in itself—and found a moment of wisdom, one of those moments India is famous for. A half-bent sign at the side of the road, in large painted red letters on a once-white background, announced "You are not stuck IN traffic, you ARE traffic."

That moment, and the mantra, has stayed with me ever since. It has helped me navigate and understand the situations we find ourselves in, as individuals and as societies, not surrounded by but creators of our "stuck-ness." The difference in perspective, in language, and in experience that define the tensions between scientists and nonscientists, between those observing the traffic, counting the cars, studying the patterns, and informing the rules, and those caught in the traffic, frustrated, caught in the herd, and feeling voiceless, is an allegory of the dynamics which are driving global networks of vaccine dissent.

While medical and scientific powers somehow expect the old rules and hierarchies to hold their ground, emotions are rising and new rules of engagement are being decided outside of esteemed institutions, new relationships are being established, and new notions of "evidence" taking hold. The public is doing their own research with Google and social media at their fingertips and growing networks of like-minded people to reinforce their beliefs, emotions, and anxieties.

This is a book born of my own personal experiences and research over a nearly 20-year period, including past assumptions that I have sometimes had to challenge. As an anthropologist having lived and worked in some of the poorest countries in the world, I did not expect to come back to the United States and Europe to witness an emerging tsunami of skepticism around one of the most tried-and-true, life-saving health interventions in modern history. What happened? How did we find ourselves stuck at a point where we had created a world dependent on vaccines, taking for granted an age-old social contract with the public for whom vaccines were as normal as brushing your teeth?

It is not that the history of vaccines is without episodes of questioning and distrust, sometimes erupting into anger and resistance. The first anti-vaccine league was founded in the mid-1850s when emotions raged in the United Kingdom against a law making smallpox vaccination compulsory. I have waded through the worn and torn pages of century-old anti-vaccine pamphlets and booklets in London archives, full of vaccine emotions—"it's not natural," "against Gods plan," and "imposing on our freedom, our rights"—not unlike some of the sentiments still heard today. On the same shelves I found a first edition of Edward Jenner's book

Vaccination Against Smallpox (1798) where, in the margins of the page describing how the vaccine works, the book's owner had scribbled angrily, "Bah Humbug!!"

Furthermore, well before the advent of social media, print and broadcast media played a key role in amplifying rumors and perceptions of risk around a number of vaccines. In 1974, an article published in the United Kingdom reported on 36 children who the authors suggested had developed neurological complications following their diphtheria, pertussis, and tetanus (DPT) vaccination.[1] The suggestion of a risk was quickly picked up on television channels and mainstream newspapers, triggering public fears around the vaccine and mobilizing the formation of an "Association of Parents of Vaccine-Damaged Children." Vaccine coverage plummeted in the United Kingdom from 81 percent in 1974 to 31 percent in 1980,[2] causing a resurgence of more than 100,000 cases of pertussis and 36 child deaths by 1979.[3] The vaccine was reassessed with more studies investigating the reported reactions, and it was deemed safe and important enough to continue its use, although anxieties remained.

Panic around the vaccine also travelled to the United States, amplified by an early 1980s TV documentary called "DPT: Vaccine Roulette" and a book, *Shot in the Dark,* also causing drops in the vaccine's acceptance. In Russia, the DPT vaccine concerns were different, partly fueled by anti-government sentiment,[4] but also triggering a 30 percent drop in DPT vaccine acceptance.

Vaccine reluctance and refusal are not new, but the viral spread of doubt and questioning today travels at unprecedented speed and reach, with many, many more vaccines and combinations of vaccines available to question. Twitter handles or Facebook pages can be powerful influencers, and, while a resource for positive change, they have also become a platform for politicians, celebrities, and other opinion leaders to instill alternative views, questions, and sometimes purposeful misinformation about vaccines.[5,6] Algorithms in the background amplify the scale and polarization of opinions while online translation tools with less than perfect translation—missing nuance and sometimes meaning—contribute to the confusion.

As this book is being written, fingers are increasingly pointing to technology companies and their algorithms as causing the contagion of vaccine doubts and fears, the manipulations of likes and dislikes, and the creation of false identities for profit or for the intentional manipulation of public sentiments.

While vaccine emotions are not immune to the manipulations of social media architects, and their schisms have become a feature of the broader landscape of public and political polarization, it is not so simple. Digital media has certainly contributed to the social amplification of risk, but there is no single culprit in this wave of dissent. Within the broader sea of questioning, there are groups purporting alternative approaches to health—nature trumping vaccines—with homeopaths and naturopaths seizing an opportunity among those losing confidence in vaccines. Other disruptions are driven by cells of stronger beliefs and ideologies—the militants—capitalizing on the unsettled state of things.

Not only has the speed and reach of information and disinformation been revolutionized by new digital technologies, power relations and social dynamics have also been dramatically transformed with groups of like-minded people—swarms—enabled to self-organize quickly, remotely, and disruptively.

Vaccines sit on the cusp of these transformations, embedded in government processes, produced by big business, innovated by scientific discovery, navigating the wonders as well as consequences of a digital revolution, supported and disrupted by local and global politics, and touching almost every human life on the planet.

As Le Bon reflected more than a century ago, we are (again) in an era of transformation, with "the ideas of the past, although half destroyed, being still very powerful and the ideas which are to replace them being still in process of formation."[7]

On the positive side, publics are engaged more than ever. They are provoking, questioning, and arguing that they are not being heard or listened to. They are making the public health and scientific community uncomfortable, making some politicians nervous, even scared, while other politicians are opportunistic, finding new constituencies among those challenging the system.

There is something in vaccines that rouses political nerves, moral and religious nerves, and sparks emotions—sometimes hope, but also fear and anxiety. Some say vaccines are no longer discussible at the dinner table given tense and opposing views, with relationships and friendships strained because of differing views on whether or not to vaccinate. At a public level, vaccine mandates provoke protest, expressions of old and new emotions against government control, while at an individual level, the act of vaccination can trigger layers of personal emotions and beliefs.

The depths of these sentiments are not unique to high-income countries. Vaccine mandates, fines, and sometimes imprisonment have been used to punish those who do not vaccinate, in even the poorest countries.[8,9] These coercive measures have provoked protests and demands for personal liberties, as well as dignity and respect.

Some communities have protested by bartering their participation in vaccination programs for other more pressing felt needs like water and electricity. Their feeling is that they are accepting vaccination for the government or international organizations, not for themselves, and they see an opportunity to voice their personal and community grievances in high-visibility vaccine campaigns like that against polio.

In April 2019, a local government representative in northwest Pakistan called for a boycott of polio vaccination until a regular electricity supply was restored. The regular interruption of their electricity was affecting their pumps and water supply, and they were not only going to boycott the polio vaccination, but part of their appeal was to "lock all the official buildings, including educational institutions and health centres in protest."[10] This is one of many protests that occurred over the decades-long polio eradication initiative, a cry to put into perspective the broader needs—and dignity—of the community.[11]

Today, we are in the paradoxical situation of having highly effective vaccines but doubting publics. While the majority still believe in vaccines, and many of those who are questioning them reject the label of being called "anti-vax," there is a growing swell of dissent. People are asking whether we really need so many vaccines. Are they safe? What are the real motives behind vaccination? Political gain? Economic gain by governments and the pharmaceutical companies? Who is the state to impose mandates on our freedom of choice and impose on our religious or other beliefs?

The debates around vaccines have become entwined with geopolitical issues, as well as political campaigns, religious and cultural issues, celebrity causes, and age-old devotion to Mother Nature over modern technology. While some people are merely hesitant yet continue to vaccinate, others are more extreme in their anti-sentiments, joining their vaccine views with other sentiments from environmental (anti-chemical and anti-mercury), to anti-government control, anti-abortion, and even anti-migration—building constituencies well beyond vaccine circles. In extreme cases, vaccines and those who deliver them have become a target of violence, such as in the killings of polio workers in Pakistan and Nigeria. And, in a new form of "weaponization," Russian bots have been found to intentionally seed divisive rumors and emotions inside online vaccine debates.[12] The research which identified the bot behavior revealed that they did not just focus on amplifying negative sentiment, but instead aimed to further polarize vaccine views—both pro and con. Of the messages identified, 43% were pro-vaccine, 38% were anti-vaccine, and the remaining 19% were neutral. This was not about the vaccine, this was using vaccines as a medium to amplify and polarize emotions to further divide society. As the researchers conclude, "this onslaught of content is meant to divide us, not just on vaccination but as a society."[13]

Alongside these changes, the ground beneath vaccine confidence has also changed. Acute levels of distrust and polarization characterizing the broader social and political environment are fertile ground for the spread of vaccine rumors and resistance, amplifying underlying grudges, frustrations, and disenchantment with the powers that be. Just as the election of US President Trump and the UK referendum vote for Brexit should not have been a surprise, vaccine reluctance and resistance have been brewing for years, but no one believed it could erupt into the levels it has. This is a public cry to say "is anyone listening?"

Waves of measles outbreaks have come and gone in the past, some more disabling and fatal than others. But what is different is the reasons for the outbreaks. Already in 2013, Anne Schuchat, then Director of the US Centers for Disease Control's (CDC) National Center for Immunization and Respiratory Diseases, noticed a trend. On a CDC Telebriefing about the measles outbreaks that year, she talked about "a story of striking contrasts" and "a very different dynamic."

"I want to tell you in particular about why they were unvaccinated," she explained, "because it's so different than what we were seeing in back in 1989 to 1991. Seventy-nine percent of the US resident cases that were unvaccinated (in 2013) had philosophical objections to the vaccine. Cases mainly occurred among people who were unvaccinated due to philosophical objections."[14]

The "very different dynamic" that Dr. Schuchat described in the United States has become a more global phenomenon. Global vaccination rates of even the oldest and tried-and-true vaccines is stagnating. While difficulties getting access to vaccines persist in some settings—particularly those rife with conflict—waning vaccination rates are additionally exacerbated by philosophical beliefs and emotions fueled by rumors.

In *Stuck*, I have chosen a focus on rumors as a valuable window on public sentiments, as an "index of morale."[15] Too often, rumors have a bad reputation, perceived to be negative or incorrect. As an anthropologist who studies rumors—how they start, what keeps them alive, and what impacts they can have—I have seen their importance as a means of seeking answers where official sources are not delivering, for collective sense-making in the face of uncertain risks, and as a beacon signaling new information of an unforeseen risk not yet recognized through more formal channels. Although they can be used in more sinister ways, stoking panic or polarization, we should take rumors more seriously. Even the more negative ones have a story to tell.

Whether true, untrue, or somewhere in between, rumors affect people's behavior—individually and collectively. Epidemics can be sparked, financial markets crashed, and political leaders overthrown "just" because of rumors. They could be a matter of life or death.

Rumors are dynamic and evolving. They live inside the webs of daily life, embellished by culture, politics, personal experiences, beliefs, and histories. They have many caretakers, each bringing their own interpretation and reinterpretation, some amplifying rumors, some quelling them. Not only does the content of a rumor change as it travels through social networks, but the environment around rumors can change, sometimes dramatically.

Rumors can thrive in some environments and wither in others. They can create a lot of noise—not unrelated to the origins of the word from the Latin word *rumorem* meaning "noise"—with little impact, or they can contain important signals of evolving information that can have significant impact. Rumors are everywhere, from the Pacific Islanders sharing their news through the "coconut wireless" to the locals in the DR Congo referring to "radio trottoir" or "sidewalk radio" as a local term for gossip or rumor spreading. Rumors thrive in situations of uncertainty and fear, such as during the Katrina disaster in New Orleans. Rumor-sharing can sometimes expose a valuable canary in the mine, providing critical life-saving information, or it can mislead people into making the wrong, even fatal, decisions.

Think of the "telephone" game where you sit in a circle and one person starts by whispering a piece of information into his neighbor's ear, and the information travels in a series of whispers around the circle until the last person has the task of announcing what he or she heard. Some call it "Chinese Whispers." It is rarely the same as how it started as, even in small circles, simple phrases can get lost in translation. The big difference is that the telephone game reveals what can naturally happen, without an intention to deceive or purposely convert your neighbor to follow a different belief.

Now imagine what happens when the motivations are different, when intentions are not to play a game, but to influence the trajectory of emotions and beliefs and to purposely misguide, to distract and divert people, and to create panic. Not only does the message change, the reaction to it changes.

The premise of *Stuck* is that vaccine rumors are here to stay, but that is not a bad thing.

I argue that rather than focusing on trying to debunk rumors, we should look at rumors as an eco-system, not unlike a microbiome. Vaccine reluctance and refusal are not issues that can be addressed by merely changing the message or giving "more" or "better" information. Debunking rumors, one rumor at a time, will not fix the questioning and convictions. It is too late for that. What is needed is a more fundamental change around the fertile ground which is fueling the concerns, rumors, and heated debates.

Rumors need gardening, perhaps weeding, but cycles of rumoring are important to reinforce social networks, share sentiments, and make sense of unknowns. It is a resource, a clarification of who are the influencers and who are the followers, and an important medium for negotiating reason and emotion in the face of uncertainty.

One of the early events that prompted me to think about writing this book was the 2003–2004 boycott of the polio vaccination campaign in Northern Nigeria. At the time, I was leading UNICEF's strategy and communication work around new vaccines and vaccine partnerships, including the launch of the Global Alliance for Vaccines and Immunization, but I found myself doing more crisis management in response to a number of countries calling for help as they faced pockets of resistance in their immunization programs. At the same time, I was getting local calls in our New York Headquarters asking why UNICEF was giving countries the measles (only) vaccine rather than the MMR vaccine—was there really a problem with the MMR vaccine, as was circulating in the press? A climate of questioning and distrust was growing (see Table I.1).

The Nigeria boycott was not triggered by any evidence of a specific problem with the polio vaccine: the resistance was about what the vaccine represented, the global powers who designed the campaign, and the central Nigerian leadership who were seen

Table I.1 ANTIVACINATION SITES ENCOUNTERED IN FIRST 10 SITES
DISPLAYED

	Search Term				
	"vaccination"		*"immunisation OR immunization"*		
Search engine	Antivaccination in first 10 sites displayed (rank order)	%	Antivaccination in first 10 sites displayed (rank order)	%
Google	1,2,3,4,5,6,7,8,9,10	100	0	0
Netscope	2,6	20	4	10
Altavista	3	10	1,5	20
GoTo	2,3,5,6,8	50	3	10
HotBot	1,3,4,7	40	0	0
Lycas	3,4,5,7,10	50	0	0
Yahoo	8,9,10	30	0	0
All 7 search engines		43		6

Davies P, Chapman S, Leask J. Antivaccination activists on the world wide web. *Arch Dis Child* 2002;87: 22–25.

as being complicit in the global effort in the eyes of local citizens who distrusted it. As many of the stories in this book reveal, vaccine revolts are a type of catharsis. They are rarely only about the vaccine, but also unleash underlying sentiments about personal and collective histories, relationships with government, big business, and international bodies. As Melissa Leach and James Fairhead poignantly write in their book *Vaccine Anxieties,* "while vaccination is easily represented as a universal, neutral good, it is actually bound up with politics: with struggles over status, authority and value."[16]

In northern Nigeria, in 2003, local rumors evolved into wider vaccine resistance when the governor of the state called for a boycott against polio vaccination which lasted 11 months. Political tensions following a northern Nigerian candidate losing the presidential election to a southern candidate converged with the other underlying reasons seeding distrust and anger that finally triggered the boycott. Rumors quickly spread that vaccines from the West were sterilizing children, particularly in light of the post-911 war on terrorism interpreted as a war on Muslims. A recent history of a multinational drug trial where a child died had also instilled widespread distrust and prompted legal suits against the drug producer. Even though the child's death was assessed as unrelated to the trial, the community won the court case for reasons of unethical practice, and community resent remained.

The Nigeria polio boycott embodied and reacted to all these relationships, a catharsis which cost the Global Polio Eradication Initiative an estimated US$500 million to recover from the negative impacts on the eradication effort.[17] Because of the boycott, undervaccination allowed the Nigerian strain of the polio virus to spread not only across Nigeria and other countries in Africa, but to reach as far as Indonesia. The annual Hajj, an Islamic pilgrimage to Mecca, became an amplifier of the virus. One Nigerian pilgrim carried the virus to Mecca, joining millions of other pilgrims for the annual mass gathering in Saudi Arabia. Crowds of co-worshippers from around the world pressed bodies in prayer, sharing not only a common faith, but the polio virus. The determined virus traveled home with another pilgrim from Indonesia.

Struck by the Nigeria experience, its global repercussions, and the broader landscape of growing vaccine questioning, I left UNICEF in 2005 to return to academia and have more time to investigate and try to understand what was driving the growing distrust. Based at Harvard University's Center for Population and Development and Clark University's Department of International

Development, I focused my research and teaching on understanding risk and rumor in global health, from AIDS to vaccines. At Clark, I was also affiliated with the George Perkins Marsh Institute, which was home to some of the early leaders in risk research, particularly around environmental risks and hazards, which was an inspiration to my thinking about public perceptions of vaccine risks. Later in the book I talk more about what some of Marsh Institute scientists referred to as the "social amplification of risk," a phenomenon highly relevant to the current vaccine landscape.

In 2009, I moved to London, where I founded and lead a research group, the Vaccine Confidence Project. Drawing from models of information surveillance to detect disease outbreaks, my team built a monitoring system to detect the emergence, evolution, and impacts of vaccine rumors. We take the pulse, monitor the rumor weather, look for brewing storms—rumors with the potential to spiral out of control—as well as map the cultural, and historical contexts where rumors are more likely to get traction. We want to see how far and how fast kernels of concerns spread, how they evolve and adapt in different cultural and political settings, and then map the overall ecology of vaccine rumors. I brought together social scientists, psychologists, political scientists, epidemiologists, mathematical modelers, and digital media analysts into the team to try to step back and look at the issue of vaccine dissent and disruption differently, as an ecosystem, tracing the connections and patterns of vaccine emotions and consequent behaviors, locally and globally.

As my research team grew, the landscape of digital media was also evolving quickly, with social media becoming increasingly ubiquitous and the viral spread of vaccine rumors, perceptions, and anxieties moving faster and faster. The rumor weather was dynamic, stormy, and ever-changing: sometimes dying out, sometimes bursting into a thunderous storm creating public panic, and sometimes retreating, but not going away, waiting for the right moment to erupt again. The character of rumors and their spread was also changing, moving away from being one-to-one Chinese whispers to being one-to-many and many-to-many in an instant.

It was clear there was an increasing amount of fiction mixed with nonfiction, with the lines between the two not always clear. Personal stories and emotional testimonies have become the new landscape of "evidence," capitalizing on the increasingly visual modes of social media, with highly emotive videos trumping dry scientific press and going viral more quickly than health officials could make sense of.

***

This is a global story, composed of many increasingly connected local stories exposing layers of trust and distrust, hopes and fears, deep-seated beliefs, and risk perceptions—all of which influence people's willingness to accept a vaccination at an individual level, but also affect the emotions and behaviors of crowds. These are not merely physically pressing crowds, such as those in mass gatherings—whether at theme parks, sport events, or religious pilgrimage sites—but instead crowds of shared emotions and belief, what psychologist William McDougall calls "the Group Mind" in his classic 1920 text.[18]

Le Bon describes this transformation from one's personal emotions to a state where those individual sensibilities become part of a "group mind." "The individual forming part of a crowd," he writes, "acquires a sentiment of invincible power which allows him to yield to instincts which, had he been alone, he would perforce have kept under restraint . . . being anonymous, and in consequence irresponsible, the sentiment of responsibility which always controls individuals disappears entirely."[19]

The phenomenon of "group think" and the contagion of emotions is a strong theme throughout this book. Although social network influences have gotten increasing attention and analysis in the era of Big Data and social media, such as the pioneering Twitter analysis by biologist Marcel Salathé,[20] overall research on vaccine acceptance has been largely focusing on individual decision-making or large numbers of individuals, but less on the dynamics and emotions of groups which have a life of their own beyond individual behaviors and sentiments.

Understanding the contagion of not just viruses but also sentiments and beliefs is crucial to the future of vaccines. As *Lancet Infectious Disease* editor John McConnell wrote in the introduction to a special issue on Mass Gatherings and Health, "To minimise health hazards at mass gatherings, it is essential to understand the behaviour of crowds."[21] Understanding crowd behavior includes understanding the web of social networks that converge and connect individuals from larger networks beyond an immediate gathering of bodies, beliefs, and behaviors.

Patterns of rumor spread—the sharing of unverified information fueled by emotions, values, and beliefs—are signaling the need for very different strategies for engaging publics. As Salathé notes, "we found that a high volume of negative tweets seemed to encourage people to tweet more negatively. But strangely, a high volume of positive tweets seemed to encourage people to tweet more negatively, too."[22]

This is not a call to throw scientific facts out the window in favor of a sole focus on emotions and beliefs. The point is that we need a more holistic, context-aware, and dynamic engagement between publics and those who develop the technologies and determine the policies and which depend on public cooperation for their success.

The stories selected for this book are by no means inclusive as the scope of relevant examples, histories, and politics would fill volumes. Each chapter draws on examples that aim to exemplify the different points throughout the book.

Chapter 1 is "On Rumor": why they matter, what sentiments they reflect, and what news they might carry. It looks at different ways that psychologists, anthropologists, and even mathematical modelers have studied rumors and how they spread. Some have focused more on the content of rumors—wedge-driving, fear-provoking, and wishful thinking—while others characterize the different personalities of those who are rumor-spreaders versus those who are vulnerable to "infection" by a rumor. Fertile ground factors—uncertainty and risk, fear, new or disturbing events, histories and politics—which can amplify rumors are also explored, looking at why the same rumor can go viral in one setting and fizzle and die in another. Finally, the dynamics of rumor spread are considered—their patterns and speed of spread—as a window on human connectedness and crowd behavior. The viral spread of rumors is, after all, not unlike the patterns of epidemics.

I argue that all of these dimensions matter: the type of rumor, the fertile ground, the spreaders, and the patterns of spread—in short, the ecology of rumors. Trying to delete or correct a rumor is missing the point. If it is deep enough in the fabric of society, it will not be easily plucked. Pushing rumors and the sentiments they carry underground may temporarily suppress, if not aggravate, those who have strong beliefs. For those trying to make sense of uncertainty through a rumoring process, feeling censored or suppressed can further alienate them and instill even more distrust in official sources. The calls for ridding the vaccine landscape of "misinformation" as a solution to the dissent is not an option. Much of the circulating information is instilling doubt, asking questions, and not overtly telling mistruths. The bigger issue is the underlying distrust, the feeling of being disenfranchised and not heard. Listening to rumors and the stories behind them can help us understand the reasons and in those lie the cues to building new and more trusting relationships.

Chapter 2 explores the fundamental emotions of "Dignity and Distrust." Vaccine acceptance is about a relationship, about putting trust in scientists who design and develop vaccines, industries that produce them, health professionals who deliver them, and the institutions that govern them. That trust chain is a far more important lever of acceptance than any piece of information. Without these layers of confidence, even the more scientifically proven and well-communicated information may not be trusted.

Among the driving sentiments behind the current waves of vaccine questioning and dissent are a sense of lost dignity and distrust. This chapter considers those who feel that they are herded like sheep, treated as if they are expected to follow without questioning, that they have no voice. Resistance to some immunization campaigns and vaccine trials has been born out of sentiments of feeling excluded and not consulted in the planning, of sensing a lack of transparency and feeling ignored when they appeal to be engaged. These sentiments of feeling unheard and not listened to have fueled the volume of voices.

Being called "ignorant" for asking a question when driven by concern for the health of their child has also contributed to the feeling of being disrespected. From another perspective, it is not only parents who are feeling their dignity is at stake, but health professionals, too, are feeling their once trusted authority has waned and is even under threat.

As one neurologist and blogger in a medical journal writes, pointing to the harsh words and name calling on all sides, the landscape has changed from one extreme where the "unchecked authority of medical experts in those days allowed doctors to trammel the rights of both patients and research subject" to an environment where doctors are rated by patients through online sites, "the same way one rates a restaurant."[23] The felt lack of empathy, the wanting of an ear who will listen, has become fertile ground for alternative voices and alternative health choices, and fertile ground for rumors.

Enter Andrew Wakefield, whose narrative embraces "parents who know best" when it comes to evidence, championing their right to personal choice while sharing his own estrangement from the scientific community with parents who feel that they, too, are not listened to.

Chapter 3 is "On Risk." Vaccine anxieties are rarely simple, and the rumors are not all wrong. Despite their success in preventing many diseases, the reality is that vaccines will always have some level of risk. Some vaccines have more risks than others, with newly introduced, less familiar vaccines being particularly vulnerable to perceptions of risk and rumor.

But vaccine risks are not the only risks that parents are considering. They are comparing vaccine risks to the risks of the diseases they prevent, many of which have become less visible and thus their risks seem even more remote. They question why they should take even a small vaccine risk when the disease is barely evident. Even when the diseases that vaccines prevent are more visible and their risks more tangible, the perceived risks of vaccines may still provoke more anxiety and reluctance to vaccinate. Juggling these uncertainties is a time ripe for rumoring, gathering pieces of information as well as opinion while trying to decide whether or not to vaccinate.

Risk perceptions are also closely entwined with levels of trust. The higher the trust, the more willingness to take a risk; the lower the trust, the higher the risk aversion. This chapter examines risks and trust, looking at trust levels in local and national government, trust in the health services and health providers, and trust in pharmaceutical companies. It also considers the social amplification of risk—when emotions around perceived as well as real risks become contagious and spread like wildfire.

Chapter 4 is on the "Volatility of Opinion." Vaccines are no longer the social norm. Publics want choice and individuals want a voice in the decisions that affect their lives—and their children's lives. Millennials, born into the boom of new technologies, were the beginning of a new era of "digital natives" with a different access to and ownership of information and self-confidence. The proactive citizen involvement in health choices, sometimes evoking a "we know better" sentiment, disrupted the age-old trust relationship between doctor and patient, health authority and citizen, and has become particularly acute in the case of vaccines. Young parents trust themselves and their own decisions more than a system they feel has disappointed them, alienates them, and disempowers their personal beliefs. This is not everyone, but the numbers who share these sentiments and who are pushing back on what is feeling like dogma rather than democracy are growing. These volatile sentiments play out differently in different settings, mediated by local politics, culture, and beliefs and influenced by personal histories and experiences. Changing relationships between citizens and science, publics and politicians, all punctuated by uncertainty, create fertile ground for rumoring—the sharing of pieces of information, making sense of a confusing landscape of fact, partial fact, and fiction.

Chapter 5 looks at "Wildfires" and how the characteristics of contemporary wildfires—burning hotter, faster, and unpredictably—are an apt window on vaccine rumors: disrupting immunization efforts, stoking fears and burning hotter, faster, and unpredictably.

Vaccine sentiments, like fires, depend on a spark, fuel, and fertile ground to spread. This chapter also explores the notion of digital wildfires, sparks of emotions spreading like contagion through social media networks. What is striking is the difference in the patterns of these wildfires in different countries: slower burning, persisting, and ubiquitous in higher income countries, while in lower income countries where vaccines are more generally accepted, vaccine scares are more locally explosive and disruptive. The different patterns and responses to these wildfires expose underlying morale and stability, trust and distrust.

Chapter 6, on "Emotional Contagion" looks at the phenomena of the viral spread of not only emotions, but also physical symptoms provoked by emotions and stress-related reactions to immunization. It is a chapter about the power of suggestion, pieces of information, visual cues that are believable enough to trigger physical reactions. The role of social media in triggering the viral spread of emotions and symptoms is also explored as a new form of contagion, more typically triggered by line-of-sight and physical proximity, rather than remotely and globally.

A series of episodes of what some call *mass psychosomatic illness* (MPI), with groups of people experiencing dizziness, fainting, twitching, and other symptoms, are described from Australia to Japan, Denmark, Ireland, Kazakhstan, Colombia, and Brazil and all related to human papilloma virus (HPV) vaccination. The Colombia story shows the power of context in shaping illness, with more than 500 girls sharing symptoms across multiple schools, all happening in one conflict-ridden, violent area of the country. Nowhere else in the country was affected. Other stories of these types of reactions, unrelated to vaccination, reveal that this phenomenon is bigger than vaccination although they disrupt vaccination programs, take a toll on trust, and cause physical distress sometimes lasting months.

The seeming dismissal of these symptoms by health authorities who insist they are not being caused by the vaccine, but instead are "psychosomatic" or "stress-related" can cause anger among those affected.

Embedded in the crowds of emotionally triggered symptoms are some who may have other underlying conditions, making the diagnosis of psychosomatic, anxiety-, or stress-related illness even more difficult to accept for those affected.

As MPI expert Bartholomew and his colleagues write, "We may be witnessing a milestone in the history of MPI where the primary agent of spread will be the Internet and social media networks. . . . It is likely, as indeed is already happening, that their illnesses will now become symbolic of wider issues."[24]

Chapter 7 is on the "The Power of Belief." The power of belief is one of the driving reasons that rumors persist. Belief is a powerful emotion and difficult to challenge with facts. It is not about facts: instead, faith, trust, and values trump scientific rationale for those whose sentiments and beliefs are deep. In a volume of essays on "Evidence," one chapter on "Evidence for religious faith: a red herring," speaks to the difference between Plato's characterization of the difference between *logos* and *mythos*. "Myth could not help you organize your society, solve a mathematical equation, or formulate a viable economic policy," the author writes. "But equally logos could not assuage human pain and sorrow. . . . If your child dies or you witness a terrible natural disaster, you do not want a logical discourse to explain what has happened. You need the kind of comfort that was traditionally provided by myth." She concludes, "if you apply the rules of logos to the first chapter of Genesis, you get bad science and bad religion."[24]

There are more formalized religious beliefs, which are largely interpretations about religious texts because most were written before the start of vaccination, but there are also philosophical beliefs. These beliefs are about lifestyle and confidence in nature over modern medicine that are challenging the public health quest for herd immunity.

In extreme cases of belief, vaccines and those who deliver them have become a target of violence, such as in the killings of polio workers in Pakistan and Nigeria. And, in a new form of "weaponization," Russian bots have been found to intentionally seed divisive rumors and emotions, enflaming beliefs and vaccine sentiments.[25]

Finally, Chapter 8, "Pandemics and Publics," reflects on risks of the next big influenza pandemic given the current state and trends of vaccine confidence. It also signals hope in the next generation, speaking up for science and reason.

With the trend of increasing access to information has come a sense of responsibility to go online and "do the research" before trusting official sources. When talking with new mothers about vaccines, some share their regret, even guilt, about having *just* listened to the doctor "without doing their own research first."

Adding to the disconnect are different notions of time between those who grew up with their smartphones of knowledge versus the "experts," whose notions of evidence involve years of research. While Twitter time creates impatience and an expectation of rapid response, scientists and health officials need time to carefully construct their response, sometimes taking so long—or not answering at all—that they lose their audience.

"It seems that the growth of social media has facilitated the development of geographically widespread communities with fixed yet indefensible opinions," one editorial in a medical journal reflected, "where hearsay is spread intensively while robust medical evidence and guidance hold little sway"[26] And Dr. Paul Offit, outspoken in his views on the Babelian discourse on vaccines laments,

"Science has become just another voice in the room. It has lost its platform. Now, you simply declare your own truth."[27]

Amid the rhetoric of enthusiasm for "public engagement" in science, it is still largely an effort to communicate scientific concepts and research findings in more creative and understandable ways and less about listening to, as well as engaging, the public in defining research agendas, in early-stage research, and in the design of delivery strategies when a new vaccine or other health technology is introduced.

The reality is that, instead, publics have mobilized themselves, empowered by new digital media to speak their unfettered views and organize themselves, and they have access to online global audiences. They *are* engaged, but on their terms. Scientists and health and government officials were not ready for what has become a tsunami of opinions, with a public critiquing science and an onslaught of alternative notions of evidence. As one UK report on "Science as an Open Enterprise" writes, "the growth of the citizen science movement, could turn out to be a major shift in the social dynamics of science, in blurring the professional/amateur divide and changing the nature of the public engagement with science."[28]

It already has.

ON RUMOR

Rumor next, and Chance,
And Tumult, and Confusion, all imbroil'd.

—John Milton (*Paradise Lost*)

Most mornings I walk to work under the gaze of George Orwell's *Nineteen Eighty-Four* "Ministry of Truth." The "Minitru"—Orwell's newspeak for the Ministry—is a towering, granite building with windows like eyes looking down at the dwarfed buildings around it. The building inspired Orwell's writing when it was home to the UK Ministry of Information, where Orwell's wife worked in the Censorship Department during World War II.

The striking tower is now part of the University of London, and my office is in the smaller yet stately London School of Hygiene and Tropical Medicine, which the tower gazes down on. Minitru, as well as the era that inspired much of Orwell's writing, reminds me daily that our current post-truth environment, littered with fake news and anecdote-as-evidence, has been here before.

The context of World War II, with all of its uncertainties and anxieties, was a ripe time for rumors to circulate. Some were driven by genuine concerns among anxious families sharing pieces of information, eager for news about their sons, brothers, and husbands on the frontlines, while other rumors were pieces of information intentionally manipulated by governments to mislead the enemy.

In 1947, Gordon Allport and Leo Postman published their classic text, *The Psychology of Rumor*, much of it inspired by their research during the war. In a lecture they gave at the New York Academy of Science in 1945, Allport and Postman pointed to rumor research conducted by themselves and others as one of the opportunities of the war.

> Although the disadvantages of war far outweigh its advantages, yet we may reckon among its meagre benefits the powerful incentives and exceptional opportunities that war gives to scientists to advance their knowledge in fields. . . . During the year 1942, rumor became a national problem of considerable urgency. Its first dangerous manifestation was felt soon after the initial shock of Pearl Harbor. . . . This combination of circumstances created the most fertile of all possible soils for the propagation of rumor.[1]

In Boston, "Rumor Clinics" were set up to mitigate war anxiety. A network of "morale wardens" searched for rumors "in taverns and on factory floors, in schools and at parties, on wharves and in stores."[2] The *Boston Herald* published a Sunday column where it countered individual rumors, even discussing possible motives behind their spread, in some cases pointing to "Axis propaganda"—not unlike the "Axis of evil"[3] rhetoric coined by President George W. Bush's State of the Union Address in 2002. The 1940s war context, though, was a very different information environment, with far more limited communication opportunities and letters mailed at snail speed. The telegraph, which revolutionized long-distance communication 100 years earlier, was able to send short messages across the sea, but personal long-distance communication was sparse.

Many would argue that Allport and Postman, along with their student, Robert Knapp, created the most thorough and foundational classification of rumor types. Knapp considered the gathering and classification of rumors to be an important "index of morale." While Postman ran the Massachusetts Division of Propaganda Research, Knapp was put in charge of rumor control for the State of Massachusetts Committee of Public Safety, where he identified four key categories of rumors: "Hostility (wedge-driving) rumors; Fear (bogey) rumors; Wish (pipe-dream) rumors; and Unclassifiable rumors."

Allport and Postman went beyond their investigation of rumor content to consider the ferment that fuels rumors. "Where there is no ambiguity, there can be no rumor,"[4,5] they write, and they put forward a "Basic Law of Rumor" stating that the intensity and spread of rumor depends on the perceived importance of the rumor multiplied by the ambiguity of the evidence. They describe this "perceived importance" not as a rational assessment, but rather as an emotional state. "At times," they write, "the relationship between the interest and the rumor is so intimate that we may describe the rumor simply as a projection of an altogether subjective emotional condition."[6] Managing rumors is about understanding and managing the emotions which drive them, not attempting to judge whether they are true or false.

Another researcher of the same era writes about the "principle of external control," recognizing that rumor spread is particularly rife in situations where the population feels that critical decisions affecting their lives are "largely out of their control."[7] The original anti-compulsory vaccine movements in the 1800s and the current resistance against vaccine mandates are expressions of frustration and anger among a public who feel that vaccine decisions are largely out of their control. They want to take back control, or at least have more of an opportunity to participate in the decisions which affect their lives and the lives of their children. This, too, is about emotion, both individual and group emotions.

In 1916, London psychologist Bernard Hart was already examining the phenomena of rumor in the context of World War I. He recognized that rumors cannot be examined in a serial fashion, individual-to-individual, because "although the transmission of a report from witness to witness is an integral part of rumour, it is not the whole thereof. It is for this reason that most of the experimental work on rumour hitherto attempted has failed to produce much illumination." Hart was a contemporary of crowd psychologist Gustav Le Bon, who influenced his thinking. "Rumour is a social phenomenon," Hart concludes. "It is therefore necessary to take into account certain psychological principles relating to the behaviour of communities, and especially of that particular kind of community which we call a 'crowd.' "[8]

Le Bon, in his writings on the psychology of crowds, talks about the key factors of anonymity, suggestibility, and contagion that drive the formation of a crowd. "Every sentiment and act is contagious," he writes, adding that "being anonymous, and in consequence irresponsible, the sentiment of responsibility which always controls individuals disappears entirely."[9] He concludes, "These same elements that drive crowd behavior fuel the spread of rumors."

In 1935, the psychologist Jamuna Prasad studied rumors following the great earthquake in Bihar, India, and he defined what he called "characteristic situations" that can lead to rumor spread. He characterized rumor-prone situations as ones which create an "emotional disturbance," are "of an uncommon or unfamiliar type," "contain many aspects unknown to individuals affected," and are "of group interest."[10] Others consider rumoring as a type of collective problem-solving while people navigate risk and uncertainty.[11]

All of these characteristics are highly relevant to vaccine rumors. Stories of children suspected to have had serious reactions to vaccines are emotionally disturbing and even fear-provoking for parents contemplating vaccine decisions. For first-time mothers considering vaccines for their infants, the experience is new, and finding answers to their questions is of "group interest" among a globally connected cadre of concerned parents. New vaccines are unfamiliar, provoke uncertainties, and are of enough interest for individuals and groups to want to know more. Old vaccines, too, are of group interest, especially when reports of suspected vaccine side effects start to circulate. This landscape has all the "characteristic situations" that create fertile ground for rumor spread. Finally, the timing of childhood vaccines coincides with a number of childhood infections and at a time when parents are particularly focused on the evolving development of their child, thus making associations with vaccines more believable and helping to fuel the contagion of rumors.[12]

While the nature and spread of rumors have been valued as illuminating important insights on human sentiment and behavior, rumors can also carry important signals of information, especially in the context of contagious diseases.

In the later years of the 1966–1980 global smallpox eradication effort, when smallpox cases were fading and the remaining ones harder to find, every rumor of a new case became important. The World Health Organization (WHO) kept rumor registers, investigating any new whisper of a suspected case of smallpox because even one case on the planet would trump eradication.[13]

In May 1980, after the nearly two-decade concerted effort, the WHO formally declared that smallpox had been eradicated. But even then, in the report to the World Health Assembly, the smallpox eradication commission urged continued rumor surveillance. "In order to maintain public confidence in the fact of global eradication, it is important that rumours of suspected smallpox, which can be expected to occur in many countries, should be thoroughly investigated."[14] Rumors mattered for the world's health.

In 1997, the WHO established a rumor surveillance network in an effort to detect real-time signals of other disease outbreaks. In the meanwhile, with the internet and digital media gaining ground, the scale of rumor reports collected expanded into the tens of thousands. Between 2001 and 2004, 1,300 of the thousands of reports were concerning enough to investigate, and 850 were confirmed as being a genuine.[15] In 2004, a rumor system was set up in the Asian region to catch avian flu rumors in local media reports and other informal sources. Of the 40 informal reports of suspected avian flu, 9 were confirmed to be true. The rumors, unverified pieces of important information, gave valuable clues to help slow the spread of a high-risk pandemic.[16,17]

***

RUMORS IN THE CONTEXT OF UNCERTAINTY

In 2014, the highly fatal West Africa Ebola epidemic prompted rumors and conspiracy theories around the outbreak: this was a disease that was previously unknown in Liberia, Sierra Leone, and Guinea. "It couldn't be real." The disbelief and denial that Ebola even existed, especially in the early months of the West Africa outbreaks, slowed down the already-too-late public health response. Publics questioned the motives of national and international bodies that imposed quarantine and insisted on taking the ill away to treatment centers from which many never returned, all of which contributed to fertile ground for the spread of rumors. In Liberia and Sierra Leone, distrust was so high that some people were hiding their sick family members so they wouldn't be taken away. Rumors literally killed.

Denial that Ebola existed in the most affected countries, distrust of local and international organizations, and visceral fear of the highly fatal disease were among the barriers to people cooperating with the needed public health measures to tame the outbreak. Distrust of the intentions of health workers was so high in Guinea that some were killed while trying to care for people and control the spread of the virus. In Ghana, two Ebola vaccine trials were suspended because of widespread anxiety that the motive of the trials was to actually give people Ebola.[18]

Over time, with concerted efforts, rumor management and community engagement, the Ebola response moved into a largely cooperative effort, and all three of the most affected countries—Guinea, Liberia, and Sierra Leone—were eventually declared Ebola-free by the end of 2015, while the panic spread to the rest of the world.

The highly fatal virus and all its uncertainties, including a lack of available treatment, prompted fears as far as the United States, where the panic was the most disproportionate to the risk. Reports circulated that parents were keeping their children at home because their school principal had been to Africa, albeit 2,000 miles away from any of the Ebola-infected areas. *Time* magazine reported that 10.5 million tweets about Ebola were sent from 170 countries between September 16 and October 6, 2014, alone. In Spain, there was national clamor following the killing of the now famous dog named Excalibur, the much-loved pet of an Ebola-infected nurse. Many called for the Health Minister to resign after ordering the precautionary, later deemed unnecessary, killing of the dog. On Twitter, a global social media movement called "Let's Save Excalibur" catalyzed almost 400,000 tweets in 24 hours.

Forbes reported that the Malaysian and Rwandan governments called for citizens not to speculate and spread unfounded Ebola rumors online, while in Vietnam four people were summoned for causing public panic by spreading Ebola rumors through social media.

While Ebola continued in West Africa, another outbreak captured global attention: Zika. The Zika virus had been quietly infiltrating Brazil since 2013, but the news of the virus spread like wildfire in 2015, when large numbers of babies were born with microcephaly to mothers who had been infected with Zika.

At the start, the cause of the dramatic increase in microcephaly was not clear. The uncertainty, anxiety, and fear were fertile ground for rumors, especially among those desperate for an answer to the question of why this happened. Why *their* child? Could *my* child be born like that? The rumors somehow helped mediate stress by sharing concerns and finding and reinforcing each other's answers to "How could this happen here?"

With no clear confirmation that the Zika virus causes microcephaly and a lack of trust in the government, all set against a background of severe economic and political crises, rumors of all kinds and origins started emerging across Brazil, moving from street corners and spreading rapidly through social media.

Among the multitude of rumors, some media pointed to a pesticide as being the culprit responsible for the microcephaly cases. Rumors in the hardest hit northeast region, though, claimed that vaccination was the cause of microcephaly: one rumor pinned the microcephaly to expired mumps, measles, rubella (MMR) vaccines.[19] Others suggested that the Tdap (tetanus, diphtheria, and pertussis) vaccine given during pregnancy was the cause.[20–22]

The rumors evolved through a process. "It's not the mosquitoes; we've always had them." "Microcephaly did not start with Zika; we've had it for a long time—something else is causing it." "The mosquito is very democratic: it bites everyone. Why are only some babies born with microcephaly?" "It *must* be expired MMR vaccines."

Even after the government announced that new scientific evidence confirmed a causal link between Zika and microcephaly, overall distrust remained high.[23] The government's dismissal of the vaccine rumors had no credibility in the eyes of the public.

The Zika- and microcephaly-related rumors circulated well beyond Brazil. A study from the Annenberg Public Policy Center at the University of Pennsylvania conducted a survey in the United States and found that 22% of respondents believed that genetically modified organisms (GMO) were the cause of Zika, while 20% thought that "bad" vaccines were the cause of microcephaly.[24]

The globalized Zika rumors also had business impacts beyond Zika and Brazil. The Indian car manufacturer Tata Motors decided the negative rumors and Zika-associated fears were even too risky for one of their newest cars, which had been named "Zica" (short for "zippy car"). They changed the name of their new car to "Tiago," chosen from a global social media and SMS contest searching for a new name. "Tiago" is a Portuguese boy's name and was chosen over the name "Civet," a cat-like mammal. The civet was found to carry the severe acute respiratory syndrome (SARS) virus, and this might also have been too risky for the car company.[25]

***

THE CONTAGION OF MMR VACCINE RUMORS

The persistence and global spread of MMR vaccine anxieties and the suspected link with autism despite all the scientific evidence to the contrary is a story of one of the most contagious rumors, one that has gone global, building new constituencies by using multiple forums and platforms and appealing to parents' eagerness for a clear answer to the cause of their child's autism. Andrew Wakefield seeded the suggestion of the vaccine–autism link with his 1998 publication and his outspokenness in its press conference. Two decades later, he continues his crusade regarding vaccine risks despite the retraction of his publication and withdrawal of his license by the UK General Medical Council. But what is often overlooked in the finger-pointing at Wakefield as being the cause of anti-vaccine sentiment is that his 1998 publication came out on the eve of the digital revolution.

Anti-vaccine sentiment had been here before, but, in the same year as the Wakefield publication, Google opened its doors. Facebook then launched in 2004, followed by YouTube in 2005, Twitter in 2006, and Instagram in 2010. Facebook had more than 1 billion users by 2012 and more than 2 billion in 2018. Citizens became emboldened with more ability than ever to access information and connect and communicate their unfettered views.

The production, reproduction, and rapid spread of vaccine anxieties went viral as never before, and Wakefield gave them a story to tell and a meme to share. "Vaccines cause autism" was a simple, repeatable confirmation of a brewing anxiety. And it easily fit in a character-limited Tweet. Even more compelling, although Twitter allowed 140 characters initially, the average tweet was 34 characters. When Twitter doubled the permitted length to 280 characters, the average length dropped to 33 characters. Short tweets get more traction. Wakefield's meme fit the formula.

Since leaving the United Kingdom and settling in the United States, Andrew Wakefield can be found standing on the steps of town halls, in churches, and reaching out to parent groups such as the Somali Community in Minnesota who were reporting high rates of autism and where he reinforced seeds of doubt about MMR links to autism, thus contributing to a decline in MMR vaccine uptake in their community. MMR vaccine coverage among Somali children declined significantly from 2004 through 2010, starting at 91% and reaching 54% in 2010,[26,27] resulting in serious measles outbreaks.[28]

Minnesota was not the only home to a Somali community concerned about the MMR vaccine and perceived risks of autism. In the late 1990s, soon after Wakefield published his now retracted *Lancet* paper, MMR vaccination coverage dropped significantly in Sweden. And among those whose concerns persisted was the Somali community. A study conducted in 2013 found that a number of Somali parents in the Stockholm area remained worried more than a decade later. Their main fear was that their child might stop speaking after being vaccinated.[29,30] Another study in Birmingham, England, found that similar fears were circulating in the Somali community there. Mothers particularly shared their anxieties that their child might stop talking or walking after MMR vaccination.[31] Along with the diaspora of people were a diaspora of beliefs—a sharing of perceptions and concerns through shared language and social networks across the world. Most striking was that overall confidence in vaccines was strong across the Somali community, but there was a particular angst around the MMR vaccine. As with other adverse events that happen around the time of vaccination, more of them are coincidental than causal. Early signs of autism start to be recognized around the same time that the MMR vaccine is normally given, when all parents are focused on first words, first steps.

Wakefield and his followers have moved well beyond, albeit not abandoning, the "vaccines cause autism" sermon.

J. B. Handley of the autism and anti-vaccine advocacy group Generation Rescue noted, "To our community, Andrew Wakefield is Nelson Mandela and Jesus Christ rolled up into one." Internet groups such as Save Dr Andrew Wakefield, the Dr Wakefield Justice Fund, CryShame, and Vaccine Resistance Movement: VRM Updates & News from the Trenches have sprung up to support his work and finance his many court cases.

He also appeals to a growing constituency of naturopathic, anti-chemical, pro-nature, alternative health audiences, sharing the stage with those who feel that his messages resonate with theirs.[32]

> The controversial former doctor (Wakefield) spoke at a "Rally for Truth" held on the steps of the Idaho Capitol in Boise Aug. 3. . . . The event, sponsored by Health Freedom Idaho, was a springboard for organizing action promoting alternative health choice in Idaho while voicing scepticism about modern medicine, including vaccinations for children, fluoride and genetically modified foods, as well as corporatism in the medical industry and the mass media.[33]

Wakefield has become a household name for those with anxieties about vaccines, affecting countries as far away as Malaysia, whose Ministry of Health issued a public statement "Correcting the Record on Andrew Wakefield" in an attempt to mitigate the growing public sentiment against the MMR vaccine. For those who follow Andrew Wakefield, he is not correctable.

Wakefield's suggestion that vaccines can cause autism has gone global, embedded into WhatsApp and Facebook campaigns and disrupting measles-rubella vaccination efforts in Southern India, as well as making it into the headlines of a mainstream Kenyan newspaper read by businessmen, politicians, and parents. The 2013 headline provoked the question, "Are vaccines making your child mentally ill?" and the article featured emotional stories of parents convinced that it was the MMR vaccine that triggered their child's autism. One mother tells her story, which concludes, "from personal experience, I believe there is a link, the reason I never allowed my second born to have the MMR vaccination."[34]

The article highlights that "four percent of Kenyans now live with autism, which translates to over 1.6 million people," implying that vaccines had a role, referring to a research paper on "Autism in Kenya and Its Prevalence." The research paper further quotes a 2007 report published by the Autism Society of Kenya which includes a list of "prevention measures," one of which recommends: "Investigate the possibility that vaccinations may have a role in the occurrence of autism, especially the MMR vaccine used for rubella, mumps, and measles. Remember that the evidence of these vaccines and other ones containing trace amounts of mercury, causing autism are still inconclusive."[35] Although the 2007 Autism Society Report seems to have been taken off the website, the 2010 paper and 2013 article are easily accessible, providing fuel for rumoring despite the reams of scientific evidence since published to the contrary.

In 2012, a viral spread of alarm followed a decision in the provincial court in Rimini, Italy, which favored parents in a suit claiming compensation on the basis that they believed their child developed autism because of the MMR vaccination. The primary evidence used to support the parents case was the Wakefield *Lancet* paper suggesting links between the MMR vaccine and autism and already debunked and retracted in 2010, and a local Italian physician who agreed with Wakefield and had his own, alternative cure for autism.[36] In a following appeal, a higher court in Bologna overruled the Rimini court decision given the lack of credible evidence. The three years between the two cases, though, was long enough to allow the rumor wildfires to spread and take a toll on vaccine acceptance. The number of tweets related to the MMR–autism controversy and the court case in Rimini increased 543% between 2010 and 2014.[37] While news of the Rimini parents winning their case against vaccines went viral, little attention was given to the decision to overturn the court ruling in 2015.

If there is one silver lining to the public questioning around suspected links between the MMR vaccine and autism, it has catalyzed the scientific and public health community to respond. The autism community has benefitted from extensive scientific research which has repeatedly demonstrated that the MMR vaccine has no relation with the cause of autism. In fact, some research has even shown that girls who had received the MMR vaccination had less prevalence of autism than those who weren't vaccinated.[38]

But science alone is not going to change the minds of those with strong beliefs. Changing fertile ground over time is another key factor in determining whether rumors thrive or hibernate, hiding like viruses until opportunities arise to reproduce and spread.[39] Underlying histories that have seeded distrust or states of political or social turbulence or conflict can create a readiness to leap on to rumors that confirm already underlying suspicions.

The viral spread of rumors and their implicit risks are increasingly studied by social scientists, mathematicians, and physicists, particularly in the context of the new evolving dynamics around social media and Big Data. Mathematicians were already exploring various models of rumor transmission in the 1960s, with some looking at patterns of disease outbreaks as being similar to the transmission of ideas. As one researcher wrote, individuals are "susceptible to certain ideas and resistant to others," vulnerable to being "infected with an idea" which can either spread like an epidemic. "Such a process can result in an intellectual 'epidemic.'" In the *Nature* paper where the researcher published his theory linking disease epidemic patterns to the transmission of ideas, he detailed out the parallels. The infectious agent was the "idea," the infective agent was the "spreader"—the author of paper, the "susceptible" was the reader of the paper, and disease-related death or immunity was paralleled to the death or loss of interest in the idea.[40] (Populations can be resistant and stop its spread.) A letter commenting on the paper referred to mathematical epidemiology and the spread of rumors, adding the importance of considering the dynamics of "the growth and decay of the actual spreading process."[41]

In 2013, researchers at Shanghai University added another feature of rumor spreading to the model: the "hibernators."[42] *Hibernation* is a key feature of rumors that seem to be managed and debunked but are only sleeping until another opportunity arises that makes them relevant and brings them back into circulation, like a virus waiting for a susceptible victim to continue its spread.

The dynamics of rumor have had a new resurgence of analysis by physicists and mathematicians in the context of more complex landscapes of fast-moving and less predictable digital communication driven by human emotions: hopes, fears, and intended disruption.[43,44]

RUMORS RESURFACE IN FERTILE GROUND

In the history of vaccines, one of the most recurring rumors—with periods of hibernation—is the fear of vaccines being used to sterilize populations. Although suspected across a range of vaccines, the tetanus vaccine has had more frequent episodes of sterilization scares given its primary focus on girls and pregnant women. "A fundamental factor driving the rumor was that the targeting of females of childbearing age was a deviation from that in other immunisation schemes, which are directed at both sexes" writes one *Lancet* article about anti-tetanus vaccine fears in Cameroon, adding that the questioning public probed, "Why farmers, who are perceived to be at higher risk than schoolgirls of acquiring tetanus, were not to be vaccinated?"

The *Lancet* authors pointed to the World Federation of Doctors Who Respect Human Life, a Belgian-based global network for pro-life doctors, as one of the sources of the sterilization concerns. The Federation, founded in Holland in 1974, with its secretariat in Belgium, has chapters in more than 60 countries committed to "legal protection for all members of the human race,[45] from conception/fertilisation until natural death."[46] When suspicions of state-led sterilization emerged, the network raised concerns. "In advice to some influential church leaders they have expressed the opinion that tetanus vaccination targeted on young women of childbearing age is not logical, and they have strengthened a prevailing suspicion that the injections contain some sort of contraceptive, which would thus be given under false pretences."[47]

The sterilization scare in the 1990 Cameroon tetanus vaccination campaign erupted into a school-wide boycott of the vaccine, where the program was being delivered. "Cameroonian schoolgirls squeezed through doorways and leapt from windows, fleeing the vaccination teams that were visiting their school as part of a campaign to decrease neonatal tetanus," wrote one team of anthropologists.[48] Other rumors emerged that one of the local beers had a sterilizing ingredient targeting the male population, again revealing the wider distrust and an underlying anxiety about population control.[49]

In one study on sterilization rumors across health programs in Africa, sociologist Amy Kaler found that most of the rumors were related to vaccines and immunization programs, dating back to the 1950s and still recurring. The rumors across multiple countries were attributed to the polio, smallpox, tetanus, and measles vaccine specifically and sometimes childhood vaccines more broadly; all were feared to cause infertility. Sometimes the sterilization rumors were not about vaccines but were tied to other government-related programs, and fears circulated that school milk, malaria drugs, and vitamins carried sterilizing agents. These rumors instead reflect a more generalized anxiety about survival and a deep distrust of the motives of the system. To those who spread and believed the rumors, it was not a matter of whether they were fact or fiction, but whether they seemed plausible and explained phenomena that that were unfamiliar, not "logical" in their cultural or social setting or experience, or that somehow confirmed already brewing suspicions. As Kaler reflects "even the most superficially bizarre rumours can be credible." It is, after all, about their believability, not the facts.

The rumors around the tetanus vaccine traveled the world, sparked by a misinterpreted research paper on a contraceptive injection and suspicions around a meeting convened by the WHO about expanding contraceptive options and focusing on "fertility-regulating vaccines."[50] These rumor seeds fell onto fertile ground in the context of growing attention to population control, including high visibility around UN regional and global conferences on population.

In May 1995, a news wire went out in Washington DC: "Fr Matthew Habiger, PhD OBS, president of Human Life International today called for a congressional investigation of reports that millions of women in Mexico and the Philippines have unknowingly received anti-fertility vaccinations under the guise of being inoculated against tetanus."

The tetanus vaccine sterilization rumors were circulated to 60 countries through Pro-Life chapters in the Catholic network—even in the absence of social media—and on July 19, 1995, the WHO issued a press release announcing that "Disturbing reports are reaching WHO from Mexico, Nicaragua, Tanzania and the

Philippines, that the tetanus toxoid (TT) vaccine has been contaminated with a substance—human chorionic gonadotrophin (hCG)—that is claimed to reduce women's fertility." The rumors had also spread in Argentina and Bolivia.

Multiple countries opposed the vaccine, including Nicaragua, where then Cardinal Obanda of the Catholic Church and a member of the local Pro-Vida group spoke out against the tetanus vaccine due to the sterilization rumors. In Mexico, the local Comite Pro-Vida accused the Secretary of Health of genocide, claiming that the tetanus vaccines contained "abortive and sterilizing substances."[51]

"These rumors are completely false and totally without any scientific basis" stressed the then director of the WHO Global Program for Vaccines and Immunization. The statement reported that the contents of the vaccine had been independently tested in Italy (in a lab chosen by the Vatican), Hungary, the Philippines, the United States, and the Netherlands, and all results were negative for the presence of any sterilizing elements.

"False rumors concerning the safety and purpose of vaccines, such as the tetanus toxoid vaccine given to adult women, may create a loss of faith in these vaccines, result in lower immunization coverage and lead to a wholly unnecessary loss of life from the diseases they effectively and safely prevent," the 1995 WHO press release concluded.

Not only did the tetanus vaccine rumors affect tetanus vaccination coverage, they affected confidence in other vaccines. In the Philippines, the mayor of Manila issued a temporary restraining order stopping the administration of tetanus vaccine, which coincided with National Immunisation Days for polio vaccination. Even polio vaccination acceptance dropped from more than 90% to 35% due to the widespread tetanus vaccine anxieties and waning distrust in the system. (Twenty years later in the Philippines, a different vaccine scare around a new dengue vaccine similarly provoked a domino effect on waning confidence in multiple vaccines. The confidence crisis contributed to a record high measles outbreak and the return of polio after 20 years of the country being polio-free.)

In 2014, the rumors resurfaced around suspected links between the tetanus vaccines and contraception, stirred by doubts around the motives behind a nationwide tetanus vaccination campaign in Kenya. In March 2014, a press statement issued by the Catholic bishops of Kenya outlined their concerns about the vaccination campaign. "We, the Catholic Bishops in Kenya are concerned about the following issues regarding the ongoing tetanus vaccination campaign: 1) There has not been adequate stakeholder engagement for consultation both in the preparation and implementation of the campaign. The Catholic Church has not been engaged unlike other public health initiatives where we have been invited to participate as a key stakeholder; 2) There has been limited public awareness unlike other national health initiatives that are preceded by a public launch where the public can ask questions; and 3) There is a lack of public information on the rationale with a background that has informed the initiative." Initially the resistance was not about the vaccine itself; this was about the motives of the campaign and suspicions around why the Catholic Church was excluded.

The Chairman of the Kenya Conference of Catholic Bishops sought answers to the following questions: Is there a tetanus crisis among women of childbearing age in Kenya? If this is so, why has it not been declared? Why does the campaign target women of 14–49 years? Why has the campaign left out young girls, boys, and men even if they are all prone to tetanus? In the midst of so many life-threatening diseases in Kenya, why has tetanus been prioritized?[52]

The Kenya Bishops did not receive an adequate response to their concerns and continued their own investigations, coming across the old suspicions of sterilizing elements in the vaccine. Finally, on November 11, 2014, this investigation prompted Parliament to order a probe into the contents of the vaccine.

On the November 13, 2014, the WHO and UNICEF offices in Kenya and WHO Headquarters issued statements similar to that issued in June 1995. "The World Health Organization (WHO) and the United Nation's Children's Fund (UNICEF) express their deep concern about the misinformation circulating in the media on the quality of the Tetanus Toxoid (TT) Vaccine in Kenya."

"The allegations are that the tetanus vaccine used by the Government of Kenya and UN agencies is contaminated with a hormone (hCG) that can cause miscarriage and render some women sterile. These grave allegations are not backed up by evidence and risk negatively impacting national immunisation programs for children and women."

The WHO HQ statement reiterated the Kenya country statement, confirming that "WHO is concerned that misinformation circulating in the media about the Tetanus Toxoid vaccine could have a seriously negative impact on the health of women and children. The Organization confirms that the Tetanus Toxoid (TT) vaccine is safe. The vaccine has been used in 52 countries, to immunize 130 million women to protect them and their newborn babies from tetanus. There is no hCG hormone in tetanus toxoid vaccines."

Nonetheless, the rumors persisted.[53] In August 2015, the Catholic bishops of Kenya shifted their target and boycotted the polio vaccination campaign. The sterilization rumors that had disrupted the tetanus vaccination program resurfaced, and the Catholic bishops now insisted that the polio vaccines be tested to make sure they had no sterilizing agents in them. Although the vaccination campaign as a whole was not stopped, the bishops had an influence on their followers. The number of parents refusing the polio vaccine doubled from the previous year, from 6% to 12% refusing the polio vaccine. Authors of the study that reported the increase in vaccine refusals concluded that although the boycott had not stopped the vaccination campaign, "if this call for boycott is repeated in future it could have some significant negative implication to polio eradication as well as other vaccination programs in the country."[54]

The Catholic bishops call to boycott the polio vaccine was not just a safety concern about the vaccine: it was a broader concern about the motives of the campaign and distrust of the international agencies who were driving it.[55] As the Archbishop of Nairobi made clear in one interview, "We are in the status where now we must be able to kind of determine our own destiny."[56] The vaccine itself was not the *real* issue. It was about self-determination, dignity, and distrust.

[2]

DIGNITY AND DISTRUST

I forgot how to think for myself
I don't understand a thing about health
I do the same as everyone else
I'm a vaccine zombie, zombie.[1]

The colorfully animated YouTube video "Vaccine Zombie," with its loud heart-beating, boot-thumping rap song, is a poignant capturing of feeling controlled, almost robotically, with no voice in vaccine decisions.

Further down the lyrics, the sentiment becomes stronger, with the language of feeling enslaved, "I always do as requested, Like the media covertly suggested . . . Don't wanna be arrested, so I don't protest it . . . like a medical slave . . . like a medical slave."

Vaccination, from its start, has always walked a tense line between personal choice and public health, between autonomy and cooperation, and those waving the libertarian flag find a welcoming home in broader movements against government control. The "Vaccine Zombie" song and its sentiments are featured on a website called "The Refusers,"[2] also the name of their band, whose core sentiments are against government control. Another song, "Do No

Harm" bemoans the tale of modern medicine having forgotten the Hippocratic oath to "do no harm."

Resistance around being controlled by government or other authorities is a dominant theme among those who question or refuse vaccines,[3] those driven by a desire to not be "watched" or spied on, counted or controlled, and expected to "follow the herd" uncritically. The notion of "herd" immunity particularly provokes perceptions of people being herded like sheep and assuming an un-questioning herd mentality, lacking autonomy, and just doing what the "system" dictates.

In the post-truth era, "sheeples" has gained new currency. The term has been used since the mid-1940s largely to refer to those who blindly follow what government says, without questioning. Vaccine-critical websites and discussions have adopted the term, appealing to those who interpret the public health mantra of achieving "herd immunity" as a way of shepherding an uncritical, "we'll do what you say doc" public to vaccinate. Some of the vaccine critics leap onto websites driven by mantras of anti-government control, spying, and surveillance, such as "The Daily Sheeple" whose slogan is "Wake up the Flock."[4]

One website featured a post commenting on the (real) news of a flock of 200 sheep running off a cliff near the French–Spanish border after being panicked by a bear.[5] The post made a parallel be-tween the sheep's herd behavior and the way government uses fear tactics to control the public.[6]

Public notions of being controlled, and a feeling of being denied voice and choice, have been the Achilles heel of immunization from its start. Some of these sentiments arise out of principle and others out of historic experiences of being controlled by authori-ties, thus instilling anxiety and distrust especially in the face of mass vaccination campaigns or mandates. The issue of public resistance to vaccine mandates will be discussed in more detail in Chapter 4, on the "Volatility of Opinion," but here it is raised in the context of feeling that personal and community dignity and respect have been betrayed, as well as instances of distrust around the motives of authorities.

Vaccination campaigns and trials in different corners of the world have been stalled or suspended because individuals and groups feel as if they were not consulted and their views not respected. Many, like the Catholic bishops in Kenya, resented being excluded and did not trust the motives of those implementing tetanus and polio vaccination campaigns. It was an issue of dignity, respect, and yearning for a voice and conversation. They were eager for an ear willing to hear their concerns and respect their role as a trusted leader in the community with insights to contribute to the vaccination campaign.

Like the Catholic bishops who felt that they had not been invited to participate in outreach, women activists in India mobilized 52 health organizations and public activists to sign a memorandum to the Ministry of Health on October 1, 2009 demanding the immediate halting of human papilloma virus (HPV) vaccine projects in two states, calling for more information to be publicly shared "within one month" and to "Open up the issue for public debate and the opinion of health groups, women's groups and other civil society members to be actively sought."[7] On the 7th April 2010, angered by the continuation of the projects and their earlier demands not met, a new memorandum now signed by 68 organization was announced in a highly publicized press conference. This time the activists claimed that girls had died following HPV vaccination, and the Indian government was pressured to suspend the projects the same day.[8]

Although investigations later found that none of the suspected HPV vaccine related deaths were actually caused by the vaccine, but rather due to a mix of other causes including drowning, malaria and a snake bite, national implementation of an HPV vaccination program had still not started at the start of 2020. Smaller local initiatives in Sikkim, Punjab and Delhi showed some promise in HPV vaccine acceptance, but persisting anxiety and doubts in the wider public reveal the long term risks of broken trust.[9]

In 2013, the Japanese government suspended their "proactive" recommendation of HPV vaccination in response to public pressure. A group of mothers, claiming their daughters had been damaged by the HPV vaccine, formed a "victims group" and mobilized a campaign against the vaccine, as well as making demands for compensation. Their daughters' symptoms were very real, but the assessment by the committee appointed to investigate the relationship between the vaccine and the girls' symptoms found no connection between the vaccine and the symptoms and concluded that the symptoms were psychosomatic reactions, angering the mothers even more. In a global symposium in 2018, where they convened parents from around the world with similar experiences, these mothers issued a statement. Among their list of grievances, one focused not on the vaccine, but on the way they felt treated by the health authorities. It was about broken trust. It read: "victims of the HPV vaccines have to endure not only physical suffering but also emotional distress . . . despite the fact that the victims and their parents consented to the HPV vaccine, based on their trust in the Health Authorities, they are now accused of being an 'anti-vaccination group.'" In the call to action, their plea was for the government to "Refrain from actions that discriminate against, or slander HPV vaccine victims."[10]

In 2015, two Ebola vaccination trials were suspended in Ghana because of rumors circulating that the trials were being planned without public consultation, as well as distrust and fears that the vaccine would spread the dreaded Ebola virus instead of prevent it, leading to public outrage and debates among scientists and parliamentarians, all amplified by the media.[11] Again, the dramatic reaction to the Ebola vaccine rumors were not merely about the vaccine, but also about the process, about a sense of not being consulted and not being told the truth.

Vaccine stance has become embedded in a mix of features which characterize who you are and what you believe, with the social acceptance of that identity also being a matter of dignity. Francis Fukuyama, in his book *Identity Politics,* writes about three dimensions of human psyche and what drives our decisions and behavior: desire, reason, and dignity. All three influence vaccine decisions, which are no longer blindly accepted from trusted experts but instead are carefully considered and questioned, a process driven by a desire for self-determination.

Health professionals, too, feel their dignity is in question and respect for their profession is under fire. They cannot understand how some people who "should know better" are saying no to vaccines. Others are themselves becoming hesitant about one or more vaccines, making the waning trust webs even more vulnerable. Some, against their scientific judgment, are bending to the requests of their patients to delay or opt out of vaccines, eager to preserve the relationship—the trust—in the face of increasing questioning.

In research reported in *Pediatrics,*[12] doctors surveyed in the United States replied that more than 90% of parents with children under 2 years of age asked to change their child's schedule, mostly due to concerns about longer term complications and "general worries without a specific concern." Despite an abundance of evidence to the contrary, perceptions about the risk of autism still persist, with 75% of parents surveyed reporting autism concerns.

Although the physicians felt that it was not in the child's best interest to delay vaccination, nearly 40% of them agreed to the parents' requests. In a similar survey in 2009, only 13% agreed to change the vaccine schedule.

The main reason the doctors decided to concede to parents was because they felt that it would build trust with the families (82%) and that the family would be less likely to look for another doctor (80%). Most of them felt that nothing they tried worked in trying to change parents' minds.

While some doctors are worn down by the numbers of questions they receive and wish they had more time to build their patients' confidence, others simply give in to parents' demands. Others fear the aggressiveness of more extreme anti-vaccine sentiment, with one Canadian doctor commenting, the "pitchforks are coming out."[13,14]

***

These disruptions have their leaders. Andrew Wakefield, notorious among most for his faulty science around the mumps, measles, and rubella (MMR) vaccine and worshipped by others as a voice of truth, has built his following by empathizing with those who feel shut out by the system, their views and concerns dismissed as being "ignorant." His appeal to their emotions has won his following. To many of them, Wakefield, too, is a "victim" whose voice was oppressed and views censored by the scientific establishment. As one concerned parent wrote to me, "Dr. Wakefield is a man of integrity and is one of the few doctors left in this world who have spoken out. . . . My son was injured by the MMR vaccine 14 years ago. Is it ethical to sacrifice the lives of many children for the sake of herd immunity? I think not. I salute Dr. Andrew Wakefield for his pioneering work."[15]

The anger of some toward their hero's loss of his medical license is captured in online comments. One person reacted to the news by implying that Wakefield lost his license because he listened to parents: "Lost his license for listening to eye-witnesses," and then went on to see that as a reflection on a break-down in society. "That statement says so much about just how demoralized our society has become, and that was 20 years ago!"[16]

Wakefield's appeal to the emotions of parents, listening to their views and giving them a sense of dignity, has won his followers. His "you know best" message appeals to his followers, who can be seen supporting him in protests, carrying signboards, "Andrew Wakefield—for listening to parents & caring about sick kids."

Young mothers not feeling respected or having their questions dismissed are more prone to be lured to leaders who empathize and listen. As one young woman explained when considering the flu and tetanus, diphtheria, and pertussis (Tdap) vaccination during pregnancy, "I asked something, it was . . . patronising . . . the attitude . . . how they came across with the answer. . . . I felt like . . . it was, kind of, like, 'well, you got yourself pregnant, so kind of deal with it and take the leaflets and just read up and do your own, sort of, investigation' . . . it kind of felt like you just got shrugged off."[17]

Dignity is a fundamental rudder of humanity. Somehow, in the rush to vaccinate and protect "the herd," respect for those feelings and beliefs has been compromised.

As theologian and ethicist Stephen Pattison aptly wrote in a commentary around the MMR vaccine debacle in the United Kingdom, "scientists must take care not to treat fear and reservation as ignorance and then try to destroy it with a blunt 'rational' instrument."[18] Parental fears and concerns need empathy, not judgment.

The 1998 publication of Wakefield's 12-child study was certainly not the beginning of anti-vaccine sentiments and movements more broadly, as is often cited, but it contributed to the perceived credibility of already circulating concerns among parents due to reported adverse events and the suspension of two MMR vaccines in the United Kingdom in 1992. Wakefield heard the growing anxieties and distress among parents who felt their children were damaged by vaccines, and he gave them some solace. Their concerns also gave support to his own beliefs, at a time when his scientific colleagues increasingly did not. Wakefield and his followers shared a common sense of alienation from the scientific establishment. The *Lancet* retraction and the UK General Medical Council's suspension of Wakefield's credentials only strengthened the conviction of those who believe in him and see him as a martyr for their cause.

It took the United Kingdom 20 years of expensive research investigating public concerns, addressing questions, and making a concerted effort to rebuild public trust to restore MMR vaccine coverage levels to the levels they were before Andrew Wakefield published his now retracted article.

Meanwhile, the debunked rumor that the MMR vaccine can cause autism continues to travel the world, now embedded in an expanded narrative that provokes distrust of authorities and dressed in a difficult-to-argue mantra championing freedom of choice and voice.

When vaccine opinions and alternative voices not aligned with scientific consensus are dismissed or shut down, as in the pulling of Andrew Wakefield's film *Vaxxed* from New York City's Tribeca Film Festival following pressure by the scientific community on the Festival's founder, Robert DeNiro, claims of censorship are invoked. To Wakefield's followers, the truth around vaccines was being suppressed, echoing the narrative in the film itself. Other groups around the world have mobilized to defend the screening of *Vaxxed* from Australia to the United States and Italy.[19]

> You may not agree with a thesis but it is not tolerable in a democratic country, to prevent the showing of a movie. . . . the Senate has become the protagonist of an unacceptable censorship . . . we present today a complaint to the Quaestors of the Senate for violation of Article. 21 of the Constitution. (Italian Consumer Group on censoring of *Vaxxed*)[20]

The freedom theme embeds the vaccine issue in a broader rights agenda and attracts followers who may not see themselves as "anti-vaccine" per se, but who believe in the more fundamental democratic right to choose. It is again about dignity and respect.

In the case of Andrew Wakefield, there was a coalescing group of parents—fertile ground—looking for a leader, someone who would listen, someone who would take their concerns seriously and be willing to stand at a podium, speak out, and believe in their evidence—their autistic child—as "living proof" of the vaccine's risks.

They found their leader in Andrew Wakefield, who embraced and gave credence to their concerns, and he has not given up. His following has grown into an increasingly global movement of parents, mostly those with autistic children convinced that their child's autism was provoked by vaccination, those who distrust "official" information or have other grievances against government. Wakefield is the archetypal leader who has honed his message to capture the mind of the crowd. As described by Le Bon, "affirmation pure and simple, kept free of all reasoning and all proof, is the surest means of making an idea enter the mind of the crowds."[21]

Increasingly, Andrew Wakefield has been invited to share the stage with homeopaths[22,23] and members of the Green Party, those who feel that his messages resonates with theirs.

Despite losing his license to practice and having his research debunked by the broader scientific community, Wakefield has continued his campaign with almost evangelical zeal, recruiting Hollywood celebrities, parents, and politicians to join his movement. He has not been shy in approaching US President Donald Trump who, according to Wakefield, needed no convincing. In an interview with *The Independent* (UK),[24] Wakefield talked about his first meeting with Trump while he was still on the campaign trail. "There were four of us representing autism and its link to immunization. He [Trump] interjected and said, 'you don't need to tell *me* that vaccines cause autism, I've seen it personally.' We went on to discuss the issue of autism in this country [US], which is said to affect one in two children by 2032 according to CDC data, if nothing is done, if nothing changes. . . . He said *if* he were elected he would do something about it."

Some leaders are overt in spreading their views and doubts, such as Trump's tweets criticizing too many vaccines and suggesting links between vaccines and autism. Others have instilled doubt through inaction, as did former UK Prime Minister Tony Blair in withholding information on whether his son had been given the MMR vaccine in 2001, at a time when the public was particularly anxious and needed a leader to help assure them. Instead, he remained silent, creating more uncertainty and doubt.

Although clearly not loved by all, both Trump and Wakefield have their champions locally and globally. An alliance between the world's most widely known—and self-promoting—vaccine critic and the elected figure to one of most powerful political positions in the world is, to say the least, an amplifier of speculated, albeit consistently unproved links, between vaccines and autism.[25]

Anti-vaccination lobbyists saw Trump as an ally even before he won the election. Shortly after the election results were known, *The Age of Autism* posted: "Now that Trump won, we can all feel safe in sharing that Mr Trump met with autism advocates in August. He gave us 45 minutes and was extremely educated on our issues. . . . Dr Gary ended the meeting by saying 'Donald, you are the only one who can fix this.' He said 'I will.' We left hopeful. Lots of work left to do."

Rightly or wrongly Trump is seen by some as "a man who can make things happen," a challenger of orthodox thinking. Trump's widely followed tweets and public statements about children becoming autistic after vaccination and calling for the end of combination vaccines because "tiny children are not horses" are a small indicator of Trump's views on vaccines—although this stance quickly changed in the face of a measles epidemic when he called for everyone to get their measles shot.

Trump's stance on science, climate change, abortion rights, and the future of healthcare in general are all cause for concern, but a viral spread of negative sentiment around vaccines can tip confidence and, for the more infectious diseases like measles, have immediate debilitating consequences.

In Texas, where Wakefield moved after leaving the UK, the trend in vaccine exemptions has been on a steady increase, with the number of exemptions up to 57,000 in 2018. This is 4,000 more than 2017[26] and up from only 2,314 in 2003.

It was their "parents know best" empathy with the public that has launched both Wakefield and Trump to their revered leader status in their respective as well as overlapping circles. Adding to Wakefield's "vaccines cause autism" alliance with President Trump, a meeting between well-known vaccine critic Robert F. Kennedy, Jr. and the president prompted rumors of a possible vaccine science advisory role for Kennedy and made anti-vaccine advocates feel even more empowered. Kennedy is most known in vaccine circles for his outspokenness against thimerosal (a preservative used in some vaccine formulas) and his role in lobbying to remove thimerosal from vaccines through negotiations around the Global Ban on Mercury convened by the UN Environmental Program.[27]

The sense of an emerging coalition among Wakefield, Trump, and Kennedy in support of their cause emboldened vaccine critics and further nurtured what Le Bon calls a "collective mind" and "a sentiment of invincible power." The book, the movie, the billboards, the Twitter handles, and the UN global reach all capitalized and inflamed perceptions of risk, thus mobilizing the worried public to speak louder.

[3]

ON RISK

I looked a bit online, about the risks and stuff. . . . I don't really think
I looked at the risk of the disease. . . . Probably should've done. . . .
We kind of felt nature must've done something right, there must be
an in-built immunity that will develop over time and hopefully protect her. And, it's not a decision that we made lightly . . . we might
regret it in a few years' time, and we felt, either way, if something
happened to her, we would regret whatever decision we made.[1]

—Kate (age 33), on why she decided
against vaccination during pregnancy

Risk is about uncertainty and taking a chance. It is about the possibility of a negative outcome, but the hope of a greater positive outcome. A danger and an opportunity. No risk, no reward.

Risk decisions are embedded in our daily lives, some made more
consciously than others. Past experiences train our reflexes in the
face of familiar risks; other risk decisions are new, made with little
previous experience and uncertain knowledge.

In considering vaccine risks, the scientific and medical community largely focus on emphasizing the significant benefits of
vaccines in reducing disease risks compared to the risks of being
vaccinated. But parents aren't always comparing benefits and risks.
Like Kate in the opening quote, they are primarily concerned about

vaccine risks: disease risks seem less apparent in their daily lives—paradoxically because of the success of vaccination.

In the process of deciding whether or not to take the risk of vaccinating or venture the risk of not vaccinating, the questioning begins. What do others think? What is the "official" guidance? What does the science say? What does my general practitioner (GP) recommend? What do my family and friends think? And, importantly, what are my own instincts, how do I *feel* about what is the right decision in the face of risks.[2] Searching "a bit online about risks and stuff" unravels a confusing mix of information and opinions, some more accurate than others, and all with rumors woven throughout.

Kate, in deciding about vaccinating during her pregnancy, "kind of felt" that relying on nature and the baby's "in built immunity" would protect her, not necessarily because the scientific evidence stacked up that way, but because that's what her instincts told her.

Risk perceptions have increasingly been recognized as being characterized by both *calculated analysis* based on reasoning and, at the same time, *experiential influences* linked to emotions and feelings. As risk specialist Paul Slovic explains, "the rational and experiential systems operate in parallel and each seems to depend on the other for guidance . . . analytic reasoning cannot be effective unless it is guided by emotion and affect." The problem, he continues, is that "proponents of formal risk analysis tend to view affective (emotional) responses to risk as irrational."[3]

Statements implying that people's feelings and concerns about vaccine risks are "irrational" contribute to their sense of alienation and sometimes anger toward "the system" and scientific elites. More importantly, those feelings have an important function in helping navigate information, as well as rumors and experiences, in order to "make sense of" whether or not it is "worth the risk." In other words, it is not a question of someone's decision being rational *or* emotional: both are at work and both matter.

> The nurse that I saw said to me . . . "when you get to a certain stage in your pregnancy . . . you can have a vaccine called the whooping cough." . . . She'd give me a leaflet to read up on it, but again, to me, that was quite a blur. . . . Then a little bit more information came. . . . I then decided, okay, I'll do the vaccine, but in my head I was still not 100% sure, but I kind of just went for it. (Lucy, age 27, on deciding about vaccines during pregnancy)[4]

Unlike Kate's decision to not vaccinate, that same process of navigating information with instinct brought Lucy to a different conclusion, and she chose to vaccinate during her pregnancy even though she was not "100% sure."

Daniel Kahneman, author of the popular book *Thinking Fast and Slow*, won a Nobel prize for his seminal research with Amos Tversky on decision-making under uncertainty. They recognized that economic decisions are not only based on calculating the costs against potential gains, but are driven by a mix of psychological factors as well. They brought together economics and psychological science to gain insights that became the basis of what is now called *behavioral economics*.[5] The same principles are also fundamental to understanding how people make vaccine decisions in the face of risk and uncertainty.

In his personal biography for the Nobel Prize, Kahneman writes about some of his early influences. "As a first-year student," he reflects, "I encountered the writings of the social psychologist Kurt Lewin and was deeply influenced by his maps of the *life space*, in which motivation was represented as a force field acting on the individual from the outside, pushing and pulling in various directions."[6]

It is the "life space"—this "force field" of family and friends, work colleagues, news and social media, and personal and social histories that act on individuals "from the outside, pushing and pulling in various directions" as they make vaccine decisions—that need more attention and understanding As Kurt Lewin characterized it, "B = $f(PE)$," which in simple terms means B̲ehavior is a f̲unction of the P̲erson and their E̲nvironment.[7] Kate and Lucy were navigating multiple risk concerns during their first pregnancy, both wanting the best for their baby in the face of often conflicting advice embedded in a sea of facts and feelings about pregnancy. What to do and not do, what to eat and not eat, and which medicines and vaccines to take or avoid were among the many push and pull factors in their life space.

What makes the decision process more complicated—whether during a pregnancy, as a young mother, or as an individual—is the reality that vaccines *do* have risks. But, they are not always the risks that people are most worried about. One of the most common circulating risk anxieties over the past two decades is the perception that the measles, mumps, rubella (MMR) vaccination can cause autism spectrum disorders (ASD). The scientific research consistently has shown that there is *no* link between MMR vaccination and autism. On the other hand, there is evidence confirming other vaccine-related risks, such as occasional febrile (fever-related) seizures following MMR immunization, which researchers in Denmark found are caused by a genetic variation in some children. They also followed those children affected over time and found that most recovered without longer lasting symptoms.[8–11]

Each vaccine has different risks and different degrees of risk. Most vaccines have the minor risk of fever and soreness after vaccination, but moderate and (rarely) severe risks can vary across vaccines. The range of possible risks are enough to nudge a mother to reach out to not only her doctor, but to family, friends, the internet, and social networks for other opinions as she navigates the process of deciding whether or not to vaccinate. In an effort to be more transparent about vaccine risks, there are a number of websites that list the various mild and more common, as well as the rare but serious, vaccine risks for each individual vaccine as well as the risks of not vaccinating.[12–14] Parents, though, generally search a wide variety of formal as well as informal sources.

In the case of the MMR vaccine and concerns about ASD, the timing of when symptoms of autism are first recognized often coincides with the time when the MMR vaccination would normally be given, thus fueling a perception that the symptoms were caused by the vaccine. Rumors of a link between the vaccine and the onset of autism were already circulating before Andrew Wakefield and his colleagues published their now retracted case study of 12 children in the United Kingdom, which hypothesized a link between MMR vaccination and autism symptoms.[15] When the suspicion was in print, and particularly when it was covered in the mainstream media, panic about the perceived risk went viral. Over the following 5 years, MMR vaccination rates in the UK fell precipitously due to heightened risk anxieties, and measles outbreaks followed due to the lack of vaccination. It took nearly 15 years to recover MMR vaccine rates to where they were before the 1998 publication. Meanwhile, autism fears went global.

In a separate paper published in an Israeli journal in 1999, Wakefield presented a graph showing steep curves of increasing autism over time using data from California and London, noting that the beginning of the climb in both cases corresponded to the introduction of the MMR vaccine.[16] But this graph and the assumptions in both the 1998 and 1999 publications were soon debunked by extensive research which followed over the next 20 years that consistently showed no evidence of a link between vaccination and autism.[17] Other large studies, one with more than 600,000 children, showed no difference in autism prevalence among those who were vaccinated and those who were not.[18-23] Instead of pointing to vaccination as the cause, the research increasingly points to genetic reasons for autism as well as some suspected environmental influences and increased age of fathers.[24,25] Newer scientific techniques have also made it is possible to see that autism is already established in the womb, long before a child is ever vaccinated.

Nonetheless, public anxieties persist. There is still ambiguity in the public mind about the causes of autism and until that is crystal clear, the perceived risks of a link between the vaccine and autism will endure. The public wants a clear, unambiguous reason for the growing number of children with autism, and debunking the rumors of vaccines being a cause without presenting a convincing alternative explanation is a non-starter.

Thimerosal in vaccines is another suspected culprit amid the perceived possible causes of autism. The mercury-based preservative was interestingly more of a US concern, while the UK embraced the "MMR vaccine causes autism" reasoning prompted by Andrew Wakefield, which gained far more global traction. There is, and never was, thimerosal in the MMR vaccines, although it has been used as a preservative in some other vaccines. The emergence of two difference perceived causes of autism—one the MMR vaccine and the other a preservative in other vaccines—is an example of a public searching for an answer to a burning question of common concern. It is what Jamuna Prasad called a "characteristic situation" ripe for rumors.[26]

The concerns about thimerosal were the beginning of increasing public attention and concerns about ingredients in vaccines—particularly preservatives and adjuvants. *Preservatives,* like thimerosal, are used to prevent vaccine contamination, while *adjuvants*—like aluminum salts—boost the effectiveness of the vaccine, but both have become targets of questioning and presumed risk. The anxieties about thimerosal emerged in the context of wider concerns about mercury-related products in the environment, including global negotiations around a UN global treaty to ban mercury. Thimerosal contains ethylmercury which, unlike the more dangerous methylmercury, is broken down and does not stay in the body. It is used in extremely small amounts in some vaccines to prevent them from becoming contaminated and to keep them safe.

But, in 1999, public anxieties about thimerosal in vaccines prompted the American Academy of Pediatrics (AAP) and the US National Vaccine Advisory Committee to recommend removing it from childhood vaccines while researchers investigated any possible risks. The recommendation was a precautionary measure to assure the safety of the vaccine because there was "no evidence of harm" in the 60-plus years it had been used as a preservative.[27,28] Instead, the public perceived the precautionary recommendation as confirming a problem, and vaccine acceptance started to drop. The decline in vaccination was short-lived, but it took a proactive trust-building effort while extensive research was initiated. Study findings repeatedly found no links between thimerosal and autism or other neurodevelopment disorders, and retrospective studies again confirmed that autism rates did not decline even after thimerosal was discontinued.[29,30]

Not everyone agreed with the recommendation to remove thimerosal. "If it doesn't cause harm, then taking it out doesn't make it safer," reflected Paul Offit, pediatrician and head of the Vaccine Education Center at the Children's Hospital of Philadelphia. "It only makes it *perceived* to be safer, which is a very different thing. So we scared people, and we scared doctors, and we scared nurses . . . the nursery had basically suspended using the hepatitis B vaccine because we'd given thimerosal a scarlet letter. They didn't get the vaccine and (some) died as a consequence. That's not the Precautionary Principle. The Precautionary Principle means you exercise caution absent harm. We caused harm."[31]

Offit's statement reflects the challenges of addressing perceived risks. In trying to calm anxieties, they can instead provoke them.

Creating environments of doubt and questioning, and thus heightening risk perceptions, is sometimes an unintended consequence of policy decisions. In some instances, though, it is an intentional strategy among those who aim to fuel anti-vaccine sentiment and polarization. While these doubt-spreaders are highly active on social media, they have a portfolio of strategies that reaches well beyond the online ecosphere.

Billboards have become one of the various tactics to provoke doubt and spark rumors. One California billboard, featuring a photograph of a large red apple, asks the question, "If an apple contained . . . " followed by a bullet-pointed listing of aluminum, mercury, formaldehyde, polysorbate 80, MSG, and animal and fetal cells, ends with the boldly written statement, "Would you EAT IT? These are in vaccines." Another billboard from the same group was posted halfway around the world, in the downtown area of Perth, Australia. This time no apple, but instead a young woman kneeling behind a pile of books, elbows on the top, and holding an open book with a questioning look. Next to her, large bold text asked the question, "Do you know what's in a vaccine?" Farther south in New Zealand, a large black billboard featuring a black and white photograph of a traditional Maori-tattooed father—keeping it locally relevant—holding a baby asks the question, "If you knew the ingredients in a vaccine, would you risk it?"—all white letters except for "risk" in red. In Italy, other billboards provoke similar questions about vaccine risks. In Pisa, the city not only famous for its leaning tower, but also its top educational institutions, a parents' movement is questioning vaccine mandates. There, a billboard states "Il rischo dell'obbligo" (the risk of mandates) and lists the numbers of mild as well as severe vaccine adverse events that were reported between 2014 and 2016. Again, provoking questions. And in a busy street in Romania, a large red billboard is less subtle, stating in large letters "Vaccines are NOT Safe! Know the risks!"

These billboards will not be influenced by new reins on social media platforms. They are not tucked into social media circles of like-minded people, but instead capture the attention of individuals, parents, and policy-makers who are passing through the streets. The billboards provoke new questions in people who may not have considered these issues before, but are now thinking twice. As Paul Slovic points out in his discussion of risks as feelings, emotions are particularly swayed by "images and associations."[32]

This global trend of stirring up questions and posing risks, instilling doubt and distrust, is fertile ground for rumors to take hold—not just the starting of rumors, but the appetite to believe and act on them. Sometimes political leaders, in an attempt to address public anxieties, have temporarily stopped vaccination campaigns or programs in the face of scientific advice to the contrary. They want to send a "we are listening to you" message, but instead they create more doubts and fuel rumors. In 1998, then French Health Minister Bernard Kouchner suspended the hepatitis B vaccination program in schools because of public pressure and suspicions that it could cause multiple sclerosis (MS), despite advice by the World Health Organization (WHO) and other scientific bodies urging him not to suspend the program given a lack of evidence of any risk of MS.[33] Instead of assuring the public, the suspension reinforced their concerns, and vaccine uptake stagnated for more than a decade, with less than a third of children vaccinated against hepatitis B in 2008.[34] In addition to government suspension of the school program, low confidence among GPs and pediatricians due to their own uncertainty contributed to parental anxieties. One survey found that 88% of GPs surveyed in France were not confident about the vaccine's safety, and more than 60% were unsure of its usefulness, with 30% not following the official recommendation to vaccinate infants.[35] The ambiguity in advice and differences of opinion between scientific consensus, health providers, and parents contributed to heightened risk concerns in a country whose overall vaccine confidence remains the lowest in the world.[36,37]

In another case, in June 2013, the Japanese government suspended its "proactive" recommendation of the human papilloma virus (HPV) vaccine against the urging of the WHO and other professional bodies that the vaccine recommendation should *not* be suspended given the lack of evidence that the reported symptoms were caused by the vaccine. Despite the global scientific consensus, the government made the ambiguous decision to stop "proactive" recommendation of the vaccine while continuing to make it available for those who demanded it. The suspension, though, was enough of a risk signal to cause vaccine acceptance to plummet from more than 70% in 2013 to 0.6% by 2014 and 0.3% by 2016.[38,39] The public were not reassured: they were scared.

Proactive recommendation of the HPV vaccination by the government remained suspended in early 2020, with vaccine update remaining below 1%. One study published in 2020 showed that the cost of the suspension meant that an estimated 24,600 –27,300 women would develop cervical cancer resulting in 5000–5700 deaths which could have been prevented if HPV vaccine uptake had been sustained at 70% or more between 2013–2019.[40]

The Philippines tells another story of a volatile political drama around a real vaccine risk that was announced a year after a new dengue vaccine had been introduced. In November 2017, a memo from the vaccine producer reported that it had identified a new risk that the vaccine may worsen dengue disease for those who had not been previously exposed to the virus. The vaccine had been launched in both the Philippines and in Brazil because both countries had serious outbreaks of dengue.[41] While Brazil managed the newly announced risk with revised guidance and training for its health staff and was able to successfully continue using the vaccine, the news of a safety risk sparked outrage and political vendettas in the Philippines. The saga exposed multiple layers of political revenge, distrust, and long-brewing anger around political corruption well beyond the scope of the vaccine risk narrative, and the dengue vaccine program was suspended. Worse, the rage turned into high-profile court cases, with accusations of "reckless imprudence resulting [in] homicide" because of a perception that the dengue vaccine was introduced into a school vaccination program with "undue haste,"[42] despite having had an extensive review and endorsement by multiple countries.

The bodies of children, some of whom had never even been vaccinated, were dug up from their graves to try to prove that their deaths were caused by the newly introduced dengue vaccine. While the risk was real, albeit rare, the vicious political attacks amplified by social media took a toll on public trust. Parents not only feared the dengue vaccine, they shied away from allowing their children measles vaccination and even deworming medicines given by the health authorities through a school-based program. Overall public trust plummeted,[43] and record high outbreaks of measles followed.

The issue of partially effective, partially risky vaccines—sometimes called "leaky vaccines"—is a challenge to public confidence. Vaccine *do* have risks, some more than others. But they also prevent serious diseases. In the case of dengue, the new vaccine was introduced at a peak period when dengue infection was rampant, filling hospital wards and killing children. The decision to introduce a new vaccine that could mitigate the spread and catastrophic impacts of such a serious disease was compelling from a public health perspective, but was bad timing in the context of political elections.

Tensions between scientific assessments of risk and public perceptions of risk are hardly unique to vaccines and have a rich history around environmental issues. The "precautionary principle," which influenced the decision to remove thimerosal from vaccines, was established in the context of growing environmental action debates in the 1970s, when politicians and government officials were navigating a tightrope between scientific advice and citizen demands.

This was also the era when the field of risk communication was being shaped and public engagement was at the fore, and some of the issues and strategies identified then are fundamental to the key vaccine debates today. Peter Sandman, one of the early pioneers in the field of risk communication, defined some key questions that characterize risk perceptions and influence decisions. While his work has been primarily around environmental risks, the field that defined the term "risk communication,"[44] Sandman's core questions are highly relevant to understanding public vaccine sentiments: "Is it voluntary or coerced?" "Is it controlled by me or others?" "Is it fair or unfair?" "Is it familiar or exotic?" and "Is it natural or industrial?" As Sandman comments, "A natural risk is 'God's coercion.' The public is more forgiving of God than it is of regulatory agencies or multinational corporations."[45]

In the context of vaccines, issues of choice versus coercion, preferring anything natural over chemical, considering whether a vaccine is familiar or new, weighing the seriousness of the disease that the vaccine is preventing, determining whether the system is fair and trustworthy, and evaluating responsiveness to questions and concerns are all fundamental questions for those considering vaccination and characterize all the uncertainties that are fertile ground for rumoring and information seeking.

In 1995, risk expert Baruch Fischoff reflected on the evolution of risk communication in its first two decades. He framed it in a cascade of leaps from "All we have to do is get the numbers right" and "All we have to do is tell them (the public) the numbers" to "All we have to do is explain what we mean by the numbers" and "All we have to do is show them that they've accepted similar risks in the past." The next leap moved to "All we have to do is show them that it's a good deal for them," "All we have to do is treat them nice," and "All we have to do is make them partners," with a final "All of the above."[46]

In the past two decades since Fischoff's 1995 publication, the scientific community has evolved even further, recognizing that it's not just about getting "our" (scientific or government authority) risk message right, but also about understanding the public's perceptions of risk.

Meanwhile, the risk landscape has changed dramatically. With citizens armed with instant access to information and opinion and the tools to connect and share in rapid fire, there has been an unprecedented "social amplification of risk" as Roger Kasperson and colleagues framed it in their work on environmental risk. These social amplification of risk factors occur in not only the technical assessment of risks, but also in the social, political, and emotional factors that can amplify the spread of risk and consequent panic. These are similar dynamics to those in Kurt Lewin's "life space" mapping of the pushes and pulls on individuals, which so impressed

Daniel Kahneman's formative work on behavioral economics. But, in the social amplification of risk framing, when enough individuals are pushed or pulled in the same direction—when individual emotions start to move crowds instead of individuals—a new dynamic emerges. The *Social Amplification of Risk*[47] has been my bible in guiding how I look at the dynamics of vaccine emotions and the evolution of rumors and risk perceptions that affect human behavior.

One of the key reasons why there will always be vaccine rumors, some more benign than others, is that vaccines will always have risks. Even with the best scientific evidence, there will still be uncertainty, and fertile ground for rumors will come and go. The challenge is in managing the rumors and mitigating purposeful scare tactics while listening for important clues that need further investigation. Building that dialogue between citizens and scientists and engaging citizens as part of the public health endeavor, rather than shutting down the conversation with seeming censorship around alternative voices, will be crucial. It's a matter of survival.

VOLATILITY OF OPINION

The Chairman said there were few questions which had given rise to more varied opinions than the subject of vaccination.

—*The Leicester Press* (UK, 1884)[1]

On January 5, 2015, an 11-year-old child hospitalized with suspected measles was reported to the California Department of Public Health. Later the same day, six other suspected measles cases were reported—four in California and two in the state of Utah. They all had one thing in common: a visit to Disneyland theme parks in southern California. By January 7, all of the reported cases were confirmed as measles, a press release was issued, and information was shared with other state departments of public health across the country. By February 11, 125 measles cases were reported across the country, with 110 of the cases in California. Thirty-nine of the cases had visited Disney parks, 34 were exposed to those who contracted measles in Disneyland, and the sources of 37 cases were unknown. The 15 cases outside California were reported in Arizona, Colorado, Nebraska, Oregon, Utah, and Washington state—all linked to Disneyland visits. Those who caught measles were between 6 weeks and 70 years old. Ten additional cases, also linked to Disneyland, were reported as far away as Canada and Mexico, and the strain of measles that sparked the outbreak was traced to the Philippines.

Twenty-four million people are estimated to visit Disney theme parks in California every year, with 400 million visiting similar parks around the world.[2] Theme parks, like other mass gatherings, provide opportune venues for viruses to spread. International visitors share not only their fascination with theme parks, passion for sports, or shared religious faith, but they can also share viruses that they unwittingly carry home.

Crowds such as those at Disneyland are a gathering of individuals, perhaps some families and friends, but overall a heterogeneous group that may or may not have much more in common than their interest in Disneyland. But the outbreak of measles sparked a new crowd, different from the physically pressing crowds within the theme park. This new swarm—a movement—felt that the Disneyland measles outbreak was a wake-up call about their own vulnerability, largely due to others not vaccinating, and they were angry. They had tolerated the vaccine skeptics and refusers for a while, but the consequences had become real. The Disneyland outbreak—at the so-called "Happiest Place on Earth"—was a highly visible platform, a stage to perform on, and an opportunity to push for making vaccination laws stricter.

Five months after the measles outbreak was declared, a 7-year-old boy named Rhett, living with his family in one of the highest areas of vaccine exemptions in California, carried a box of more than 30,000 signatures to Governor Jerry Brown. Rhett had his own story to tell and his own emotions that motivated him to make a personal appeal along with others in support of the Senate bill (SB-277) proposed in response to the Disneyland outbreaks. The bill called for suspension of the personal belief exemption to opt out of school vaccination. In the California State Assembly, Rhett told the story of his personal fight with his blood cancer, of his undergoing chemotherapy and receiving multiple drugs and more than 50 lumbar punctures to "get the bad [cancer] guys out." He was making an appeal for parents to vaccinate their children to protect his own and others' lives because they were not able to vaccinate themselves because of a medical condition.

The State Assembly passed the bill, which was enacted in January 2016.[3] The successful overturning of the California state personal belief exemption reignited the emotions of those who had strong objections to vaccination and had used the exemption clause to waive their children's required vaccinations. Across the United States, an outbreak of demonstrations against the SB-277 legislation erupted, espousing sentiments against "medical tyranny"[4,5] and demanding freedom of choice. But the bill stayed intact.

Kindergarten vaccination rates in California climbed from 93% to 95% in the first 2 years after the bill became law, but this was alongside a worrying trend of a 250% increase in medical exemptions. Not surprisingly, these new medical exemptions were in areas that previously had the highest number of personal belief exemptions before such exemptions were banned by the SB-277 legislation.[6] New concerns emerged about doctors bending the rules and writing medical exemptions for some parents intent on not vaccinating.[7] Alongside continuing public protests against the vaccine laws were the silent ones, willing GPs accommodating vaccine dissent.

The fraudulent medical exemptions sparked a further reaction. In early 2019, State Senator Richard Pan made a case for a new bill—SB-276—calling for an additional layer of state approval for medical exemptions.[8,9] A doctor's letter would no longer be enough to evade vaccination. Emotions grew stronger on both sides.

In the midst of debates around the proposed SB-276 exemption legislation, another measles crisis was raging, with more than 1,200 cases across the country. It was the largest US measles epidemic in 25 years, and more than 700 university students in Los Angeles alone were put under quarantine to control the spread.[10] Despite the seriousness of the outbreak, protests against the proposed SB-276 bill erupted, with some arguing that the new legislation would be an extreme and unfair measure. Robert F. Kennedy Jr., outspoken in his views against thimerosal in vaccines, teamed up with actress Jessica Biehl to personally lobby against the bill at the California Senate House, but to no avail.

On the other side of the country, in Rockland County and Brooklyn, New York, another measles outbreak was spreading like wildfire through the Orthodox Jewish community, where measles vaccination rates were too low to protect the community and the virus sickened more than 400 people. The measles virus there was imported from travelers who had visited the Ukraine, the Philippines, and Israel and unknowingly came home infected to spread the virus among those who were not vaccinated in their communities.

Given the intensity of the outbreak, Rockland County took the unprecedented step of calling for emergency measures forbidding any unvaccinated person from going into public places—schools, shopping malls, restaurants, and places of worship—or risk imprisonment.[11] Although the order was only for 30 days, it was overruled as a breach of Constitutional law.

Measles also went viral in Brooklyn, where the New York City Health Commissioner put out an order that all children and adults in the most affected neighborhoods had to get their mumps, measles, rubella (MMR) vaccination or risk a fine of $1,000. A group of Brooklyn families challenged the order but lost the court case. The judge ruled in favor of the New York City's Health Commissioner's order.[12] This had become a serious emergency.

The large numbers of children who were unvaccinated were not due to religious sanctions against vaccination, but were due to concerns seeded in part by a mother from the community who founded a group called Parents Educating and Advocating for Children's Health (PEACH). The group had been active since 2014,[13] but only became more visible when serious measles outbreaks in late 2018 brought attention to the level of under-vaccination in the community. The group produced brochures, and a "Vaccine Safety Handbook" claiming to be "An Informed Parent's Guide," which tells the tale of a mother who used to trust her doctor and had her children vaccinated, but then faced a series of problems that she attributed to the vaccines. The story goes on to say that the doctor assured her that the vaccine was not the cause of her children's ear infections and other symptoms, but she decided to do her own research, only to discover a deep online archive of negative information about the safety of vaccines.

The "Safety Handbook" is illustrated with a cartoon in which a young mother is holding her baby and asking the doctor whether he had ever read *PEACH Magazine,* to which he retorts "All the references are fabricated! Throw it in the garbage!!" and the caption under the cartoon reads "Or, you could decide for yourself." A parody of itself, the cartoon portrayed a message that likely touched other mothers who felt the same dismissiveness from a doctor, provoking their drive for self-determination.

The PEACH materials, like billboards, reached beyond those searching online for vaccine information, or sharing concerns in social media circles. In addition to being available online, they were also distributed as printed brochures and a 42-page guide to members of the local community in New York, as well as mailed to Orthodox community members in other states, raising the ire of those who support vaccines, but making others think twice.[14]

Back in California, in the midst of fiery debates around medical exemptions, the governor signed SB-276 into law. But not without more protests. As the *Washington Post* headlined its story, "California governor signed a pro-vaccine bill into law this week. Then the protests got weird." Protesters disrupted the signing, with one throwing menstrual blood on the senate floor from the balcony while calling out, before she was arrested, that it was to honor the dead babies killed by vaccines. Inside and outside of the State Capitol, protesters swarmed, two chaining themselves to one of the entrances to block access. The protests continued through the week, including a candlelight vigil for all the children they believe were harmed—or killed—by vaccines.

The protesters carried signs that read, "Welcome to Nazifornia" and "This is the new civil rights movement," while singing "We Shall Overcome," thus provoking resentment from those who saw the protesters as largely white and elite.[15] The suggestion of being a civil rights movement seemed "borderline racist," as one California Assemblywoman commented, adding that "the whole conversation around vaccinations is actually one about privilege and opportunity."[16]

***

Vaccine opinions have become volatile, are exacerbated by a broader environment of populism and polarization, and are further fueled by divisive echo chambers of social media sentiment.[17] This is a perfect storm of sparks, fertile ground, and amplifiers in the form of heads of state, Hollywood and Bollywood celebrities, rogue scientists, and other key influencers using social media platforms as public podiums, writing books, making movies, and posting billboards all challenging scientific experts and health authorities and presenting alternative notions of the truth.

The characteristics attributed to those citizens who align with populist leaders and who carry emotions of anger, alienation, and resentment toward elites are not unlike the sentiments of those who are questioning and sometimes refusing vaccines. These volatile emotions have become even more entrenched with the ubiquitous use of the term "anti-vax" in the media as well as in public fora. By dividing the world into those framed as being against vaccines— from their mandates to their contents—pitted against those who are "pro" vaccine, vaccine debates themselves have become populist in nature, disallowing alternative, plural views and pitting values against science, rather than embracing both. As one hesitant but not "anti-vax" mother expressed on a BBC radio program, "We are not flat earthers!"[18]

Standing up for rights to freedom of expression, choice, and individual dignity are all healthy characteristics of democratic societies. But contrarian views are problematic for a technology like vaccines whose success—at least for many vaccines—depends on "herd" or population cooperation to reach herd immunity. Herd immunity, sometimes called "community immunity," means that enough people in a population have been vaccinated against a disease and become "immunized" so they interrupt the spread of the virus, such as measles, and protect others in the population from becoming infected. This is particularly important for people with medical conditions who cannot be vaccinated, who are too young to be vaccinated. When populism and polarization drive a wedge into the heart of democracy, and vaccine decisions are politicized, immunity suffers.

Publics in different corners of the world are challenging what has become "normal." They are tired of feeling instructed by what they perceive as finger-wagging experts and authorities. They feel alienated from the "system" and anxious about more and more vaccines, and combinations of vaccines, being recommended and sometimes required. Some are also harboring anger and frustration at the medical and scientific community's defensiveness around vaccines, which sometimes seems devoid of human emotion. Some see a political opportunity in this growing polarization, while others see a new following and a potential market for their alternative health solutions.

The United States is not alone in facing public debate. In June 2015, as Rhett was speaking to the California State Assembly, a young boy named Pau became the focus of attention in Spain. In this case, after nearly 1 month's hospitalization in intensive care, Pau died of diphtheria. His parents had refused vaccination. It was the first case of diphtheria in Spain in 29 years, and the first case in 32 years in Pau's home region of Catalonia. His parents felt deceived by the anti-vaccine sentiments and misinformation they had heard.[19]

From polarized debates around school-mandated vaccination in the United States to Australia's "No jab, no pay, no play" legislation that withdraws financial support for daycare if children are not vaccinated, tensions are running high between those pushing for personal vaccine choice and those angered that their children are being put at risk by their unvaccinated peers.

Measles outbreaks across Europe, with more than 20,000 cases and 35 measles-related deaths in 2017,[20] triggered new vaccine mandates in Italy and France. In both cases, they increased the number of vaccines required for school or daycare entry, in some cases imposing fines on those parents choosing not to vaccinate their children. These stricter laws incited protests on the streets of Italy and France among those fervent in their convictions on the right to vaccine choice, and the vaccine debates around compulsory vaccination leaped onto political campaign platforms. Unlike the populist-driven debates in Italy, the French vaccine debates prompted an improbable union between "the far-right nationalists and the far-left ecologists"[21] in a shared stance against vaccine mandates. The 2017 decision to put a mandate in place in France was not a knee-jerk reaction to the rising tide of measles cases but was a tipping point following a succession of vaccine scares, waning public confidence, and drops in vaccine uptake that prompted the government to call for a public consultation. As one commentary in the journal *Vaccine* reflected, "in August 2015, only weeks after having stated that 'vaccination is not up for debate,' then Minister for Health Marisol Touraine made what appeared to be a complete U-turn and announced that a citizens' consultation would be organized in order to find a way to restore trust in vaccines."[22]

The convergence of outcomes from the open consultation and a legal case where parents had won the argument that they should not be obliged to give their child combination vaccines which included more than the three vaccines (tetanus, polio, diphtheria) mandated at the time left the government with the choice of purchasing separate vaccines or mandating all of them. With the waning availability of older separate vaccines and the risk of waning vaccine acceptance, making all 11 vaccines compulsory seemed the best option. The choice of a mandate was also in sync with the consultation, which concluded that compulsory vaccination was the right choice at least until vaccination rates caught up and protected the public. Although debates followed, with some criticizing the process, the mandate was enacted and, by 2018, vaccine coverage started to improve.[23]

In Italy, the political dynamics told a different story. In 2017, Italy's populist MoVimento Cinque Stelle (M5S or the Five Star Movement) catapulted the vaccine mandate issue to high visibility in their political platform. The newly elected Five Star party vowed to override the compulsory vaccine legislation put in place in late 2016 by the previous Health Minister Beatrice Lorenzin under the center-left Democratic Party.[24] Anti-vaccine sentiments were particularly pontificated by Matteo Salvini, the outspoken deputy Prime Minister and lead of the League (*Lega Nord*) which shared anti-vaccine sympathies with the Five Star Movement. "Ten obligatory vaccinations are useless," he fear-mongered, "and in many cases dangerous, if not harmful."[25]

The rhetoric against vaccines drove Walter Ricciardi, the head of Italy's National Health Institute, to step down over the populist party's "anti-vaccine stance,"[26] comparing the sentiments of the Five Star Movement's Deputy to Trump's anti-vaccine ranting bemoaning too many vaccines.[27,28] Riccardi's resignation also followed the Italian Health Minister Giulia Grillo's surprise announcement that she was sacking the entire Higher Health Council (CSS).[29] The CSS is a panel of 30 scientific and technical advisors to the Ministry of Health, none of whom she had met since her appointment. Her announcement merely said "we are the #governmentof change" and it was time for something new.[30] An unsettling change-for-the-sake-of-change, alongside flagrant dismissal of scientific evidence.

It took a massive measles outbreak to stall the Five Star attempt to abort the compulsory vaccination legislation. By early 2019, compulsory vaccination was in place after a roller coaster of debates and volatile opinions. Fines up to US$560 could be imposed for unvaccinated children sent to school, and those under 6 years old would be sent home.

The Five Star Movement was founded by the highly popular actor and comedian Beppe Grillo. In 1998, he was already spreading his skeptical views on vaccines. In a crowded theater in Milan, he strode up and down the aisles, waving his hands as he stirred the audience. "The principle of the vaccine is to take a healthy child, not even 1-year old, with a perfect immune system. . . . Then you inoculate a small little virus so that he gets used to it a little bit. If a big virus arrives, the small little virus has been running for years and it F**k$*! the big one. . . .

"But, if the big virus does *not* arrive, the little virus stays there, stays around. And beside him there is also some mercury. . . . Then the small little virus passes into the immune system, and we have no more immune defences."[31] Grillo then projects a chart on the screen and claims that the rates of infectious diseases have been manipulated to persuade people to believe in miraculous vaccines (already evoking the sentiments of "fake news" before Trump made it part of his daily vocabulary).

Grillo sermonized his view that diseases have not disappeared because of vaccines, claiming instead that they are cyclical and go away by themselves. His parting words in his one-man show, "Soft Apocalypse," pointed to multinationals as the real cause of our illnesses.

These planted some of the early seeds of doubt and popularized the anti-establishment views of Beppe as the 2009 co-founder of the Five Star Movement, along with his web strategist partner Gianroberto Casaleggio. In the "MoVimento Cinque Stelle" title "a capital "V" for "Vaffa" ("f—ck off"), vaccines, and vaccine mandates feature largely in the category of issues that are deemed to be "hands off" to the establishment and left to the choice of "the people."

Grillo's profile was not unlike Trump's in his crude language and flagrant disregard of science, aided (initially) by his own Breitbart web strategist and having what Uri Friedman aptly called his "mythical link" to the public.[32] Add to that his pre-election anti-vaccine tweets.

Vaccine resistance fits perfectly into populist agendas. It is an exemplar of what populism is all about. One analysis of the links between vaccine confidence measures and populism in Europe found significant correlations between the proportion of the electorate voting for populist parties and the percentage of people who reported low confidence in the importance, effectiveness, or safety of vaccines. The study goes as far as concluding that "popular distrust of elites and experts that seems to inform vaccine hesitancy will be difficult to resolve unless its underlying causes—an iniquitous economic system and unrepresentative political system—are addressed."[33] In short, focusing on building vaccine confidence in the context of health services is not enough. The issues are deeper. Concerned publics feel they have no voice and no choice in decisions that affect their lives, alienated from "elites," and treated merely as numbers not as people with opinions and emotions. The concept of "medical populism," coined by social scientist Gideon Lasco, describes the conundrum of vaccine resistance well. He writes, "medical populists are willing to break taboos and disrupt conventions of the medical establishment by provoking conflict and casting doubt on established medical conventions."[34]

Those who claim to represent "the people" can, like Trump, come from exactly the background he defies. As political scientist Cas Mudde points out in an interview in *The Atlantic*, it's not about living a similar life, but about claiming to share the same values that leaders leverage to identify with "the people." "Someone like Donald Trump, who clearly is not a commoner, can nevertheless pretend to be the voice of the people. He doesn't argue, 'I am as rich as you.' What he argues is, 'I have the same values as you. I'm also part of the pure people.'"[35]

From Italy's Five Star party to Poland's Law and Justice party (PiS), Trump, Brazil's far right populist Jair Bolsonaro, Turkish President Recep Erdogan, Joko Widodo in Indonesia, and India's Hindu-nationalist Narendra Modi,[36] us-versus-them intolerance is back on the rise. It is "the people" versus the political and financial elites, with medical and scientific experts seen as among those who are deemed elitist, speaking a different, inaccessible language and entwined with big business and pharma as well as politics.

In Poland, a citizen's bill calling for a stop to compulsory vaccination was led by a group called "Stop NOP" (meaning "Stop Adverse Events" in Polish). Stop NOP has strong allies in the Polish Parliament, particularly among more right-wing populist members who also supported a campaign against in vitro fertilization and the closing of borders to refugees. The group's website features information from anti-vaccine groups in the United States that are claiming vaccines can cause autism and other side effects as its rationale for stopping mandatory vaccination, reflecting the global connectedness of these movements.

In June 2019, Stop NOP organized its third "International Protest Against Mandatory Vaccination—Warsaw and the Whole World." In the previous 2 years, it had mobilized thousands to walk through Warsaw with banners calling for "medical freedom."[37] By 2019, the network had grown. Between May and September 2019, coordinated global protests took to the streets in a sequence that moved from Italy, to Canada, Poland, Ukraine, Bulgaria, Russia, Uruguay, New York, Washington, Croatia, and Germany. Although the numbers were small in some of the protests, the global connectedness was telling. Outside of the mothership Warsaw Protest, which featured Andrew Wakefield, Germany reported the largest numbers.

This was not Wakefield's first visit to Poland. He addressed a Naturopathy Conference in 2017. At the 2019 protest, though, he focused on vaccine risks and his mantra that "parents know best," prompting loud applause from the crowd.

Standing on the steps of a city square in front of the protest crowd, Wakefield applauded the gathering for standing up for "health freedom and resistance to coercive and dangerous vaccination practices," the driving refrain of the rally, then he amplified the scale of vaccine risks into a "worldwide tsunami." He criticized "men in white coats" who "protest the need to maintain herd immunity to protect the vulnerable while being paid a bonus for every fully vaccinated child" and then invoked the importance of trust (having been one of the "men in white coats" who was a breaker of public trust). "When that trust is gone all that is left is force . . . and forced medical procedures are a disgrace and they are an admission of failure.

"People of Poland *must* have control, must have dominion over their bodies, and those of their children. Parents know what is best for their children and they have *always* known that. Mothers *must* trust their instincts and the world will be a safer place."

These populist-like chants reached out to "the people" with empathy, while scorning medical elites and damning coercive vaccination, which he carried on to say don't work and aren't safe anyway. While criticizing authorities of not telling the truth, Wakefield preached his own false narrative, but it was what his followers wanted to hear, all translated in real time by the Polish moderator.

Beyond the live preaching to the crowd in the town square, the sermon was amplified by social media. The YouTube video with Polish translation was viewed nearly 40,000 times.

The Stop NOP movement is having an impact as the number of vaccine refusals in Poland has increased from 4,000 in 2010 to an estimated 40,000 in 2018.[38] Similar sentiments circulate on social media and through Polish diaspora networks, showing influence on vaccinating behaviors such as among Scotland's Polish community, where vaccine acceptance has also been declining after having been a community known for high vaccination acceptance.[39,40]

These are not new emotions in the context of vaccination, especially around the issue of free will. Immunization, since its beginning, has always been poised on a tense line between individual rights to choice and societal rights to health, between rights and responsibilities—the right to choose, with the caveat that your choice does not harm others.

In the United Kingdom, public outrage followed the first compulsory vaccination act in 1853, and emotions were further inflamed in 1867, when the mandate was extended up to 14 years of age.[41] While the new legislation initially resulted in more than 90% vaccine acceptance, anti-vaccine sentiments and growing public protests undermined the legislation and vaccination rates dropped to 3%.

Leicester, England, was home to one of the most vibrant anti-vaccine movements, and the 1867 expansion of the mandate was the tipping point that triggered the establishment of the first Anti-Compulsory Vaccination League in 1869. The UK movement grew, along with other movements in Europe. Protests in Stockholm led to a drop in vaccination to as low as 40% in the city, but they had less effect on the rest of the country.[42]

In England, multiple cities were engaged across the country, but Leicester attracted the largest crowds.

On March 23, 1885, the "Great Demonstration" took place. After a carnival-like procession, 80 000-100 000 people gathered in the marketplace bearing banners with slogans such as "Keep your children's blood still pure" and "Stand up for liberty" or the picture of a skeleton vaccinating an infant's arm held by a grinning policeman. The climax was the motion, passed by acclaim, that "The principle of Compulsory Vaccination Acts is subversive of that personal liberty which is the birth right of every freeborn Briton."

This was, after all, the era of John Stuart Mill's classic work *On Liberty*, published in England in 1859. Important to the context of the vaccine resistance movement is the environment of broader libertarian sentiment which Mill captures well in his introduction. He writes, "there is a considerable amount of feeling ready to be called forth against any attempt of the law to control individuals in things in which they have not hitherto been accustomed to be controlled by it."[43] In Poland, where "principles of freedom" were enshrined in their independence from a previous dictator state, emotions around freedom from state control transferred to freedom from mandated vaccination, perceived as state-controlled. "In our past," one colleague told me, "we did what our leader told us to do. With our independence from the old regime, people see vaccine choice as part of that new found freedom."

As with many episodes of vaccine resistance, context and history are key to understanding what is driving the dissent. The 1853 and stricter 1867 compulsory vaccination acts hit a nerve amid already brewing emotions against government control and in support of personal liberty.

In 1884, the *Leicester Press* reported, "The parents and burgesses of Leicester passed a resolution expressed 'heartfelt satisfaction' at Alderman Stratton's outspoken defence of parental rights against believers in vaccination and the medical despotism which is aiming to acquire control over every household in the country." In the same year, the *Leicester Mercury* published an article on an anti-vaccine demonstration which captured the depth of the anti-vaccine convictions.

> By about 7.30 a goodly number of anti-vaccinators were present, and an escort was formed, preceded by a banner, to accompany

a young mother and two men, all of whom had resolved to give themselves up to the police and undergo imprisonment in preference to having their children vaccinated . . . three hearty cheers were given for them, which were renewed with increased vigour as they entered the doors of the police cells.[44]

In reaction to the public protests against the compulsory smallpox legislation, a Royal Commission was established in 1896 to investigate the complaints. While the report concluded that vaccination was important to protect the public, according to Swales's historical account, "in a gesture to the libertarian cause it recommended the abolition of repeated penalties."[45] The government, also sensitive to the prevailing libertarian emotions and swelling public dissent, not only abolished the repeated penalties, but additionally established in 1898 what became the first legal "conscientious objector" vaccination exemption and the first use of the term "conscientious objection."

The revolt against the smallpox vaccination mandate in the United Kingdom also struck libertarian nerves in the United states, and, in 1882, the New England Anti Compulsory Vaccination League was established. Three years later, a New York City Anti-Vaccination League followed. Not unlike 21st-century vaccine resistance, those protesting mandates in the 19th century were "middle-class citizens who didn't trust government, science or medicine," and they hailed from large cities, were educated and earned a decent living.[46]

[5]

WILDFIRES

"We've taken an ecosystem that was sustained by fire," said Dr. Finney, "and turned it into one that is destroyed by fire."[1]

In 2009, a "mega-fire" raged across the southern state of Victoria, Australia, consuming more than 2,000 homes and 450,000 hectares of land. It was named "Black Saturday," after the date when the fire sparked and spiraled into its unprecedented trail of destruction, estimated to have caused more than US$4 billion in damages.[2] Following an extreme heat wave a week earlier, "tinder dry" land, and high winds, the state was on alert for fires. But the extent of the flames and their devastation was beyond expectations.

Prompted by Black Saturday and the pattern of increasingly intense wildfires around the globe, 90 scientists and experts from 20 countries and a range of disciplines gathered at Florida State University in 2011 to examine what was driving the dramatic change in not only the scale and intensity of the fires, but also the change in their fundamental nature.[3]

The trend continued, and, in the summer of 2018, California battled the highest number of wildfires on record.[4] Washington state also faced severe wildfires burning faster and more furiously than previously experienced and prompting the governor to declare a state of emergency.[5] "Big fires burn differently than small fires," physicist Mark Finney told the *New York Times*, "[these] wildfires often exhibit nonlinear behaviour or act counterintuitively. . . . As it [the wildfire] gets bigger, it burns fuel at a higher rate, and that means they are a lot less predictable than we thought."[6]

A year later, bushfires across Australia set a new record. Between September of 2019 and January 2020, CNN reported that 17.9 million acres of land had burned, killing 28 people and millions of animals across six Australian states—"an area larger than Belgium and Denmark combined." The report compared the scale of the devastated landscape to the California wildfires where 247,000 acres burned in 2019 and 1 million acres in 2018.[7]

These fires were different. It was no longer about calling on more resources to put the fires out; it was time to reexamine what was driving them.

Wildfires, and particularly their changing nature—burning hotter, traveling faster, and following less predictable paths—struck me as an apt assessment of the current state of vaccine skepticism and distrust of those who produce, regulate, or recommend vaccines. The emotions are burning hotter, traveling faster, and their paths and populations are less predictable. It is, like unpredictable wildfires, a situation of "radical uncertainty" as economists have termed the "extreme events that (can) happen but had not previously been imagined."[8]

As Pankaj Mishra reflects in the *Age of Anger*, "History is far from being repeated, despite many continuities with the past. Our predicament, in the global age of frantic individualism, is unique and deeper, its dangers more diffuse and less predictable."[9]

Social media and smartphones are ubiquitous in even some of the most remote corners of the world. Rumors, anxieties, and emotions can spread like wildfires, clustering around shared sentiments, making them look even more ubiquitous than they really are, and sometimes triggering behaviors that most individuals would not have dared on their own.

In January 2019, the governor of Washington announced another state of emergency, but this one was not due to raging wildfires. Measles, a disease the United States had eliminated in 2000, was back with a vengeance and reached emergency proportions. It was particularly bad in Washington state, which has one of the highest rates of unvaccinated children (along with other states in the Pacific Northwest, home to a strong anti-vaccine movement).

One news report told the story of a young mother in Clark County, the most affected area, who was too frightened to take her 8-week-old son outside the house. He was too young to be vaccinated, and his mother knew that vaccine refusals were common— as common "as being vegan or going gluten free."[10] Nearly 25% of the county's children did not have the needed vaccination.[11]

What was happening in Washington state was an echo of outbreaks across the world. In 2018, the measles wildfires across the European region alone escalated to nearly 83,000 cases and 72 deaths in both children and adults.[12] The total was more than double the number of measles cases across all of Africa in the same year. In 2019, the measles fires continued, escalating to 300% more cases in the first 3 months of 2019 than a year earlier. The World Health Organization (WHO) called the state of outbreak of measles "alarming."[13] The state of vaccination was ailing.

***

DIGITAL WILDFIRES

The attacks of 11 September 2001 revealed that States, as well as collective security institutions, have failed to keep pace with changes in the nature of threats. The technological revolution that has radically changed the worlds of communication, information-processing, health . . . and allowed individuals the world over to share information at a speed inconceivable two decades ago. . . . [O]pportunities for cooperation are matched by an unprecedented scope for destruction.

—UN General Assembly 2001

In 2013, the World Economic Forum's annual *Global Risks* report highlighted the risks of "digital wildfires in a hyper-connected world." "Digital wildfire" was one of the three key case studies presented in the report, where the authors warned that "the global risk of massive digital misinformation sits at the centre of a constellation of technological and geopolitical risks." While recognizing the benefits of new technology, they stress that "hyper-connectivity could enable digital wildfires to wreak havoc in the real world."[14]

It already has. Havoc has emerged in financial markets, publics, politics, and polities. The World Economic Forum's 2019 Global Risk Report identified "media echo chambers and 'fake news'" as one of the top 10 global risks.

Media echo chambers and fake news are the tip of the iceberg when it comes to the risks inherent in the digital landscape. Physicist Neil Johnson, in his analysis of online hate,[15] exposes "network of network" dynamics not unlike those connecting vaccine questioning and vaccine-angry groups. Johnson points to interconnected clusters that "form global 'hate highways'" that "cross social media platforms, sometimes using 'back doors' even after being banned, as well as jumping between countries, continents and languages." Although "hate" is not the dominant emotion in the vaccine resistance movements, strong emotions of anger and betrayal drive the growing connectedness and pave a "global highway" for online emotions around vaccines.

Hyperconnectivity has also fueled undue panic in public health, driving behaviors that can accelerate rather than mitigate the spread of infectious diseases. The risk of digital wildfires in a hyperconnected world is particularly relevant to the growing constellations of vaccine skeptics and their impacts on global health. New digital technologies and their algorithms can fuel social media swarms and emotional contagion with unprecedented speed and scope. Rumors, anxieties and fears can spread like wildfires, clustering around shared sentiments —making them look even more ubiquitous than they really are, and sometimes triggering behaviours that most individuals would not have dared on their own.

In early 2017, WhatsApp and Facebook posts spread across the southern states of India instilling doubt and anxiety around a measles-rubella vaccination campaign. The southern states typically have the highest vaccination rates in the country, but this was different. The campaign aimed to vaccinate more than 35 million 9-month to 15-year old children across five states, but it was disrupted by a social media storm fueled by a mix of conspiracy theories, safety concerns, and rumors that the vaccination was intended to sterilize the Muslim minority population. In Tamil Nadu, the campaign only reached 35% of those who were meant to vaccinated.[16]

Social media-saturated urban areas had higher rates of vaccine refusal, while private schools posed another challenge, with parents reporting anxieties about the safety of and even need for the vaccine. Concerns ranged from autism fears to perceptions that the vaccine had been banned in the United States and sent to India instead.

A year later, the same rumors sparked emotions through another WhatsApp campaign in the Indian state of Uttar Pradesh (UP), causing several Muslim schools to refuse the vaccines. The *Times of India* featured one headline on the disrupted immunization program claiming, "WhatsApp rumours make 100s of UP madrassas reject vaccination."[17] In some cases the *madrassas* (Koran schools) did not allow health officials to enter the school, while others encouraged students to stay home on vaccination days due to rumored fears that the vaccines caused infertility. While some Muslim leaders tried to change the narrative and assure the public that the rumors were not valid, anxieties remained.

These rumors echoed polio vaccine sterilization rumors which had circulated in Uttar Pradesh in early 2002. The fears then were around the motives of Western countries supporting the global polio eradication effort, but who were also engaged in a post-9/11 war on terror, sometimes interpreted as a war on Muslims. The difference in 2002 was that there was no Facebook or WhatsApp. The internet was commonly pointed to as to "the source" of the rumor, although most villagers had never used a computer.

In January 2019, a new vaccine panic erupted across Mumbai schools with social media wildfires spreading rumors that the vaccines were a plot by the government to sterilize Muslim children.[18] These rumors swirled in social media storms in the southern states in 2017, then in northern Uttar Pradesh in 2018, before travelling to disrupt the Mumbai vaccination campaign. The rumor narrative fit well with the pro-Hindu, populist discourse of the Narendra Modi government, which only got stronger on the heels of an election, with anti-Muslim sentiments intensifying around the India–Pakistan border.

Each of these social media wildfires not only sparked fear and emotions, they disrupted vaccination efforts. In Mumbai, only 50%

of those who were expected to be vaccinated actually got the vaccine, with mostly Muslims missing out.[19]

The use of social media to spread false news, provoke anxiety, and incite fear is hardly unique to manipulating vaccine views. In the context of India's political elections, social media campaigns and political trolling were being used and abused widely to reach large populations across India. One Indian news article aptly described political trolling as "the act of using emotions, lies, false accusations and broken logic to undermine your opponent and win an argument in a political arena. This often involves twisting various sources, such as religion, to look like they say that your views are right."[20] The same rules govern the vaccine disrupters—twisting truths, appealing to emotions, and provoking panic.

As the editor of the eye-opening volume *Empires of Panic* conclude, "Governments and state agencies around the world are increasingly focused not simply on mitigating the 'real' threats posed by natural disasters, pandemics, conflicts, and financial crashes, but equally on handling and allaying virtual anxieties."[21]

Science writer Laurie Garrett, captures a poignant example of handling "virtual anxieties" in an article in *Foreign Affairs* on "The Real Reason to Panic About China's Plague Outbreak."[22] She writes,

The Chinese government's response to this month's outbreak of plague has been marked by temerity and some fear, which history suggests is entirely appropriate. But not all fear is the same, and Beijing seems to be afraid of the wrong things. Rather than being concerned about the germs and their spread, the government seems mostly motivated by a desire to manage public reaction about the disease. Those efforts, however, have failed—and the public's response is now veering toward a sort of plague-inspired panic that's not at all justified by the facts.

The Chinese government had deleted a WeChat post shared by a doctor working in Beijing's Chaoyang Hospital describing the condition of a couple who had come to the hospital with breathing difficulties and high fevers. While presumably trying to avert panic by not sharing clear information, the government prompted more fear and anxieties spread through Weibo and other platforms.

Philanthropist Pierre Omidyar's Democracy Fund, alarmed by the unintended consequences of new digital media, launched an investigative report asking the burning question "Is Social Media a Threat to Democracy?" Their premise: "Fundamental principles underlying democracy—trust, informed dialogue, shared sense of reality, mutual consent, and participation—are being put to the test by certain features and attributes of social media; they have disrupted our public square."[23] Every one of these principles is entwined with the waning state of vaccine confidence. The public square has been disrupted.

Cosmologist and astrophysicist Sir Martin Rees has written extensively on risk and the future of the planet, and he similarly reflected on the hazards of social media in an interview about his book, *On the Future: Prospects for Humanity.* "I think we're going to have growing problems of governance," he reflected, "because, obviously, with social media, everyone is more engaged, panic and rumor can spread literally at the speed of light. It's going to be very hard to make the right balance between privacy, security, and liberty when we're in a world where a few people—by error or by design—can cause a disaster that can even cascade globally. This is something that is really new and that's a real tension for governance in every nation."[24]

Facebook itself has acknowledged the challenges and potential perils of its own platform. "As unprecedented numbers of people channel their political energy through this medium," their Civic

Engagement manager admitted, "it's being used in unforeseen ways with social repercussions that were never anticipated. If there's one fundamental truth about social media's impact on democracy, it's that it amplifies human intent—both good and bad."[25]

Political scientist Larry Diamond warns against hubris around the potential of new technologies in writing about "liberation technology" and its vision of new modes of citizen engagement and political voice, as well as its use as a means to facilitate social and political movements. He reflected on the 15th-century invention of the printing press, which was an enabler of the Renaissance, the Protestant Reformation, and the Scientific Revolution but also "facilitated the rise of the centralized state and prompted a movement towards censorship." The telegraph, too, was "hailed as a tool to promote peace and understanding," but "what followed was not peace and freedom, but the bloodiest century in human history."[26]

Larry Diamond's calling out the risk of hubris around the potential of new technologies echoes sentiments in the World Economic Forum 2013 *Global Risks* report. The 2013 report points to another type of hubris around medical science, posing the question whether "modern medical successes bred a sense of hubris—excessive confidence that science will always come to the rescue?"[27] The case of vaccines is a poignant example of a modern medical success where excessive confidence in the technology has overlooked the vulnerabilities it depends on—from public trust in governments and reliance on big business, to assumptions about societal cooperation. Add to these vulnerabilities the risks of digital wildfires, when new "liberating" technologies are instead used to undermine rather than support vaccination. In May 2018, people refusing the polio vaccine doubled to 70,000 during a vaccination campaign in Karachi, Pakistan.[28] Their fears had been stoked by a falsely titled video clip circulating on mobile phones and claiming that 16 children had died following polio vaccination.[29] The challenge in this episode, and emblematic of the evolution of rumors, is that it started with a "grain of truth" but evolved, spreading like wildfire as the story changed.

Three months earlier, in another city 275 kilometers away from Karachi, three children had died following measles vaccination. The local authorities claimed the deaths were likely due to expired vaccines. The story was featured on the television news, showing ambulances and a crowd of mourning relatives outside the hospital where the children had died. To stir panic in the context of the polio vaccination campaign months later, someone had taken clips of the earlier televised report and the images of grieving families and reedited it with headlines that 16 children had died from polio vaccination. The video went viral, and vaccine refusals skyrocketed.

The coordinator for the polio program in Pakistan's Sindh Province, where the incidents took place, told *The Telegraph* (UK) that "Social media is kind of one big phantom which we have never been able to be on top of."[30]

In April 2019, a panic around polio vaccination swept northwest Pakistan following a video posted on Facebook claiming that the polio vaccine was poisoning children. France 24 reported from Islamabad that vaccine refusals soared to 10,000 per day, much higher than the 200–300 refusals during the last campaign,[31] and children in multiple cities were rushed to the hospital.

The mass hysteria exemplified the risks of digital wildfires, particularly in situations of heightened anxiety. In the same week, one polio worker and two policemen assigned to guard polio workers were shot dead by militants, further contributing to the uncertainty and fear.

Hostility to immunization teams flared last week after religious hard-liners in the city spread false rumors, raising a scare on social media that some children were being poisoned and dying from contaminated polio vaccines.

The rumors spread like wildfire, triggering mass panic in northwestern Khyber Pakhtunkhwa Province. Mobs burned a village health center, blocked a highway, and pelted cars with stones. Medical workers were harassed and threatened.

Mosques made announcements that children were having cramps, vomiting, and diarrhea after they were given "poisonous" polio drops. Word went out on social media that some children had died. Panicked parents rushed their children to hospitals, overwhelming health authorities. In Peshawar alone, about 45,000 children were brought to hospitals complaining of nausea and dizziness. Officials described it as mass hysteria, asserting there had been no deaths confirmed.

"The mistrust in one segment of society, that refuses vaccinations due to religious beliefs, is translating into the rest of the country, which is something not seen in the past," said Babar Atta, the government's top coordinator in the drive against polio.[32]

Three months later, a young mother in Karachi was divorced by her husband after she betrayed his instruction not to vaccinate the children. The 26-year-old mother had welcomed the polio vaccinators into their house to vaccine the children while the husband was at work, having also had the children surreptitiously vaccinated against other diseases without his knowledge. The husband was convinced that the vaccines were not safe, persuaded by the toxic rumors that the vaccines were dangerous.

These social media-driven rumors can not only drive panic and disrupt local wildfires of dissent, they also can spark mimicry in distant countries, provoking equally damaging disruption.

On September 22, 2017, a case of monkey pox was reported in an 11-year-old boy in Southern Nigeria.[33] A few weeks later, rumors spread "like a wild fire in a *harmattan* season,"[34] as one local news source reported, claiming that the army was coercively injecting school children with the monkey pox virus. Panic went viral, and parents ran to the schools, demanding to take their children out and causing the schools to close to calm the chaos.

> The incident that occurred on Wednesday, October 11, will remain a lasting memory in the minds of many school children, their parents and teachers in the South-East geopolitical zone for a long time.
>
> Parents and guardians had dropped their children in their various schools in their usual routine and left for their places of work for the day and had looked forward to picking them up after school. But around 10 am that day, there was commotion in the zone. Through the social media, information began to spread that some people in Army uniform had invaded schools in the region and were injecting pupils with Monkey Pox virus for the purpose of depopulating South-East and South-South. Parents rushed to their children's schools and demanded to take them home.[35]

The monkey pox outbreak in the region was real, with 42 cases additionally confirmed after the 11-year-old boy. There was also an ongoing army operation to deliver health services in the area, but it did not include vaccinations or other injections, and the health services were being offered in the Catholic Church and not in the schools.

The fears and panic triggered by the rumors fed on widespread distrust and anxiety in the community, which is plagued with drug wars and gang-related violence, as well as on a recent shoot-out in a local Catholic Church which killed 12 people. There was enough history to make the rumors believable.

One month later, the Nigerian scare was mimicked in Madagascar. In November 2017, a plague epidemic was raging in Madagascar[36] infecting more than 2,000 people and killing more than 140 during the 4-month outbreak. On November 8, rumors started circulating claiming that school children were being forced to have a plague vaccination without their parents' consent,[37] echoes of the phantom monkey pox injections rumored to be given to Nigerian school children.

As the rumors went viral on social media, panicked parents ran to the schools to get their children out. As one local newspaper reported, "stones were pelted at teachers and furniture was strewn everywhere as furious parents rushed to collect their children, concerned about the validity of these vaccination. . . . One parent allegedly exclaimed: 'Are you trying to kill my child or what?' "[38]

There was no vaccine against the plague, and no forced vaccination in the schools, but the context of uncertainty and fear was fertile ground to make the rumor seem believable, and parents panicked.

The power of social media to allow these fear-provoking memes and strategies to quickly jump countries and continents is unprecedented. In a different episode of transnational mimic behavior, a 5-year-old girl's body was exhumed in South India in her parents' effort to prove a vaccine had caused her death.[39] The South India story mirrored the narratives of stories circulating online and in social media about children in the Philippines who were being exhumed from their graves to investigate their cause of death because of suspicions that they had died because of the newly introduced dengue vaccine.[40] These were not routine procedures. The timing of these rare events was no coincidence.

***

In early 2018, Facebook was confronted with a flood of lawsuits over breach of data privacy while also being called on to restrict hate speech, bullying, and other violent or offensive content on their platform. Calls were also coming for other technology giants to clean up the harmful misinformation about vaccines, calling them out one by one: "Think Facebook has an anti-vaxxer problem? You should see Amazon."

US Congressman Adam Schiff wrote to Facebook's Mark Zuckerberg and Google's CEO Sundar Pichai asking, "What actions do you currently take to address misinformation related to vaccines on your platforms? Do you accept paid advertising from anti-vaccine activists and groups on your platforms? What steps do you currently take to prevent anti-vaccine videos or information from being recommended to users, either algorithmically or as a suggested search result?"[41]

The CEO of the American Medical Association sent a letter to a longer list of Silicon Valley CEOs making a similar appeal: "we urge you to do your part to ensure that users have access to scientifically valid information on vaccinations, so they can make informed decisions about their families' health."[42]

In the United Kingdom, the Secretary of State for Health and Social Care also called for algorithmic purging of online anti-vaccine messages, although recognizing the risk of this being perceived as censorship and something that could backfire.[43]

To address the growing rage, Facebook and other technology companies vowed to create stricter online rules, community guidelines, and standards, and put a sea of moderators to work to keep harmful content in check.[44] News headlines featured the moves of different tech companies to put the clamps on vaccine disinformation: "Pinterest Blocks Vaccination Searches in Move to Control the Conversation," "YouTube Yanks Ads From Anti-Vaccination Conspiracy Channels."

"Twitter's knee jerk reaction is to purge," remarked David Carroll, an associate professor of media design at the New School, in pointing out the ethical tightrope. "What it does is erase history in an almost Orwellian way."[45]

How have vaccine sentiments landed in the same league as hate crimes, Arab Springs, and other riots? While these platforms are certainly amplifying the fires of dissent and discontent, they cannot be blamed for the underlying emotions. These emotions will find another outlet if suppressed until the day the deeper issues are addressed.

The real challenge is that many of the vaccine narratives, both pro and con, are embedded in websites or social networks whose primary focus is on other issues. Accidental and intentional misinformation are only part of the thread of conversations. There are also websites solely devoted to challenging vaccines, pushing for free choice, or promoting a vaccine-free childhood, many of which also propose natural health solutions. Even these websites have become sophisticated in their choice of names and their narratives, which make them sound very open and parent-friendly, intending to support "informed decision-making," yet clearly having a strong bias against vaccines, which only becomes apparent after reading further down the pages and following the rabbit hole of hyperlinks.

Even then, where is the line between causing harm and breaching the right to freedom of expression?

As one headline announced, "Facebook's plan to kill dangerous fake news is ambitious—and perhaps impossible"[46] YouTube's CEO Susan Wojcicki similarly summed it up in an interview with the *Financial Times* by saying, "it's not like there is one lever we can pull and say, 'Hey, let's make all these changes' and everything would be solved. That's not how it works." Former chief information security officer at Facebook Alex Stamos raised one of the various challenges in a separate interview. "You can't moderate content unless you see it. You can't find the bad guys unless you are collecting data about them."

Physicist Neil Johnson pointed to the limits of focusing on individuals rather than stepping back and looking at constellations of behavior. "Most of the approaches to dismantling the online support are at the individual level," Johnson shared in an interview with *The Atlantic*. "They always seem to want to find the bad guy, the needle in the haystack, the ringleader. What our work shows is that is not the way to go. . . . You try to catch one fish; will it stop the grouping? No, of course it won't. Fish number three becomes number two, number two becomes number one. . . . So you need this systems-level approach or you'll never understand this behavior."[47]

While tech companies scrambled to figure out ways to put limits on harmful content without breaching privacy and allowing legitimate freedom of expression, the UN Office of the High Commissioner for Human Rights launched a major report on the role of governments and companies in ensuring the right to freedom of expression and access to online information.[48] The UN Special Rapporteur urged states to "reconsider speech-based restrictions," arguing that "human rights law gives companies the tools to articulate their positions in ways that respect democratic norms and counter authoritarian demands." In short, don't let authoritarian states abuse tools to limit harmful content as a means to interfere with the broader right to freedom of expression and access to information.

***

When I first started reading about social media platforms being asked to police their content on everything from hate speech to anti-vaccine content, all I could think was, "Are we just shooting the messenger rather than dealing with the source? Do we *really* think the anger, dissent and proselytizing missions of those trying to convert others towards a 'vaccine-free' life will just go away if their podium is moved? Why should the messenger take the bullet?"

It reminded me of the news about the killing of nine health workers delivering polio vaccination in Northern Nigeria in February 2013. Three radio journalists were arrested and a radio station's license was suspended for hosting a program where the presenter spoke out against the polio vaccination campaign and its ties with the West as well as questioning the safety of the vaccine. The journalists' arrests and the suspension of the license to broadcast was attributed to the claim that the radio program "incited" the violence that led to the killing of the health workers.

There were no reported arrests of those who actually killed the health workers, only the arrests of the amplifiers of negative sentiment. I was troubled by the reaction, the seeming dismissal of the culprit and displaced blame. But can we really disentangle any single event or piece of information from the societal, political, and technological context in which it occurs? In the course of researching and writing this book, it has struck me that the biggest glaring cause of the tsunami of vaccine protests is the fact that the medical and public health community are so focused on the act of vaccination, of counting, of reaching numerical targets that efforts to engage the web of society, culture, politics, and economies that surround that vaccination has been lost.

In 1964, Marshall McLuhan introduced his well-known "the medium is the message" concept in his book *Understanding Media: The Extensions of Man*. He recognized that the message, or content, cannot be separated from the medium in understanding its impact. "The 'message' of any medium or technology," he writes, "is the change of scale or pace or pattern that it introduces into human affairs. The railway did not introduce movement or transportation or wheel or road into human society, but it accelerated and enlarged the scale of previous human functions, creating totally new kinds of cities and new kinds of work and leisure."[49]

McLuhan quotes Pope Pius XII, who was concerned about the implications of new media already in 1950, "It is not an exaggeration to say that the future of modern society and the stability of its inner life depend in large part on the maintenance of an equilibrium between the strength of the techniques of communication and the capacity of the individual's own reaction." This is truer now than ever.

The world is not new to cycles of history crying for a recalibration in consideration of new technologies, new processes, and their implications for society, politics, economies, and the environment. In 1982, a powerful film called *Koyaanisqatsi* (a Hopi term translated as "life out of balance") provoked viewers with slow-moving films of landscapes, cityscapes, traffic patterns, and contrasts, all set against the eerie and disquieting music of Philip Glass. It was the first of what became the "Qatsi Trilogy," released in 2013 and more relevant now than ever.

Reggio, the filmmaker, echoes McLuhan's point of not separating technology from content, from life. He writes, "these films have never been about the effect *of* technology, *of* industry *on* people. It's been that everyone: politics, education, things of the financial structure, the nation state structure, language, the culture, religion, all of that exists within the host of technology. . . . It's not that we *use* technology, we *live* technology. Technology has become as ubiquitous as the air we breathe."[50]

Individuals around the planet are "living" new technologies now more than ever. Social media is ubiquitous even in the remotest, poorest corners of the globe. It has enabled as well as disrupted social life, it has had an impact on production, on knowledge sharing. It has allowed and disrupted democracy, and while being an asset to health surveillance and data sharing—even telemedicine—it has taken an unexpected toll on global health.

Two hundred years ago, Mary Shelley published her riveting tale, *Frankenstein; or, The Modern Prometheus*. It was a tale of hubris, of fascination to know more and more, of man creating a monster and then abandoning him, leaving him to find his own way. But, having neglected his creation, Dr. Frankenstein is faced with unanticipated revenge by his creation. Shelley's novel was one of the earliest, if not the first, science fiction novels, presenting insights on the human condition and the struggle that arises with the desire to know more and more, yet unprepared to deal with the consequences.

We are increasingly confronted with the risks and consequences of social media and global connectivity. The algorithms, bots, and trolls that live behind the screen are manipulating and polarizing emotions, fears, and alternative truths, undermining public trust in science. Findings that Russian bots and trolls have become embedded in the vaccine debates not to undermine vaccines, but as a platform—a Trojan Horse—to further destabilize democracy should be a clarion call to re-tame the creation that has become, in some ways, our own worst enemy.

EMOTIONAL CONTAGION

By participation in the mental life of a crowd, one's emotions are stirred to a pitch that they seldom or never attain under other conditions. They are, as they say, carried out of themselves, they feel themselves caught up in a great wave of emotion, and cease to be aware of their individuality.

—William McDougall, *The Group Mind* (1920)[1]

In May 2014, in the northern rural town of Carmen del Bolivar, Colombia, 15 girls aged 11 to 17 years, were admitted to the local hospital with symptoms of shortness of breath, tachycardia, and numbness in their arms and legs. They were all from the same school. At first, the symptoms were suspected to be related to food, water, or possibly pesticide or iron poisoning. Then, suspicions started circulating that this was a reaction to the human papilloma virus (HPV) vaccination that all the girls had received 2 months earlier.

In the coming weeks, 75 girls from the same school showed similar symptoms, and eventually more than 500 girls in the area reported symptoms of numbness, dizziness, nausea, difficulty walking, and, for some, full body spasms. Local news media showed the girls being carried to hospital emergency rooms, and images of the girls experiencing twitches, convulsions, and fainting went viral on YouTube. Many of the images mimicked similar YouTube videos circulated by girls and their mothers in the United States, Denmark, Ireland, and Japan—all following HPV vaccination.

A medical team was sent to Carmen de Bolivar to investigate the cases, but after reviewing all the information and conducting laboratory tests, nothing could explain the symptoms. The reports acknowledged that the girls were ill, but the only plausible explanation was mass psychogenic illness (MPI) provoked by anxiety around the HPV vaccination and possible underlying stress in a region affect by a history of violence and abuse unrelated to the vaccine.

In an attempt to calm panic and anger around the events, the President of Colombia made a public statement that the girls' symptoms had been investigated and were found to have no organic link to the HPV vaccine. He announced that this was a mass psychogenic reaction due to fears of the risks of HPV vaccination. As the President gave his address, the Minister of Health was boarding a helicopter to meet with the community in a town hall gathering in Carmen de Bolivar. By the time the helicopter landed, instead of being welcomed by the community, the Minister was met with a crowd of angry protesters and the army had to be called in.

The girls, their parents, and the local population saw the diagnosis as humiliating and insensitive. The presidential message, which was intended to calm the public and show empathy with the girls' illness, instead backfired and caused public outrage around the idea that this was "just" a psychological reaction.

In spite of public outrage, with citizens claiming that the vaccine was responsible for the reactions, the government stood by the scientific evidence and maintained full support for the national HPV immunization program. Nonetheless, HPV vaccine uptake declined dramatically with public mistrust spilling over to other vaccines and decreasing uptake of vaccines unrelated to HPV.

In August 2017, 3 years after the event, 700 individuals filed a class action suit against the Colombian government and the vaccine producer, all claiming vaccine injury.[2] Meanwhile, the YouTube videos of the dramatic reactions among the Colombian girls continue to circulate, subtitled or with voice-overs in different languages and seeding vaccine rumors and anxiety around the globe.

One video "Fue el Guadarsil" ("Guardasil did it"), opens with a sepia-toned image of a Dylan-like Colombian guitarist, harmonica around his neck. In Spanish subtitled in English (to reach as wide an audience as possible), he strummed his guitar, singing an ode to his sister Cara: "Tell your mother, tell your sister . . . When Cara was vaccinated she was feeling well, she was buried yesterday. . . . " The camera moves from the guitarist to a group of girls lined up in rows facing the camera as the guitarist appeals, in his mourning voice, "Don't let them vaccinate you, because it can kill you. . . . Don't let them vaccinate you, because it can kill you." The way the girls line up in rows, almost military-like, with stern faces looking into the camera, mimics images in a series YouTube videos which started in Japan and then jumped to Denmark, Ireland, and on to Colombia.[3]

The Colombia outbreak was the most dramatic case in a series of episodes of mass fainting, twitches, and related symptoms following HPV vaccination, echoing scenes from the 2014 film, *The Falling*.

Soon after Colombia introduced the HPV vaccine, nearby Brazil introduced the vaccine into a school program for 11- to 13-year-old girls. The first vaccination rounds went well, with more than 85% of the eligible girls being vaccinated. But trouble started in the second round, when 80 girls had symptoms similar to those reported in Colombia—headaches, dizziness, fainting, and weakness. News of the symptoms spread quickly through social media, as well as in print and broadcast news. Even though most of the girls fully recovered from what was diagnosed as anxiety reactions, the episode instilled fear, and HPV vaccine acceptance plummeted to 45%.[4] The Colombia panic had spread.

Australia was one of the first countries to introduce the HPV vaccine, and the first to experience these anxiety reactions. In 2007, 25 girls attending a Catholic school in Melbourne, Australia, started feeling dizzy and nauseous, some with headaches, one with palpitations, another with hyperventilation. While the symptoms varied, they all had one thing in common: their first HPV vaccination.[5] Most of the symptoms resolved, and the girls reactions were short-lived, but media reports went viral, causing a panic around the HPV vaccine. Australia's HPV vaccination program recovered from the reactions and the country now has one of the most successful HPV programs. Japan, however, had a very different experience, one that paralyzed the HPV vaccination program for years.

In Japan, the HPV vaccine was introduced in 2009 and widely accepted with nearly 80% uptake. However, in March 2013, 50 girls made the news with vivid images of being rushed to the hospital with twitches, involuntary movements, headaches, and fatigue after receiving the HPV vaccination.[6] A movement of mothers emerged claiming that their daughters were "damaged" by the HPV vaccine. They organized a National Network of Cervical Cancer Vaccine Victims and mobilized an aggressive public campaign that captured mainstream media and paralyzed the government. The movement influenced the Japanese parliament—the National Diet—and tied the hands of the Ministry of Health.

The government appointed a committee to investigate the reported symptoms following vaccination, but no clear cause was found and no evidence of a link between the vaccine and the reported symptoms. The conclusion was that the reactions were psychosomatic, further fueling anger. Court cases were launched by parents blaming the government for their daughters' symptoms. Meanwhile, research in Japan and internationally continues to show the effectiveness of HPV in preventing HPV-related cancers, and studies find that the symptoms suspected to be caused by vaccination are happening at the same rate among teenagers who have not been vaccinated.[7,8]

June 2019 marked 6 years of the Japanese government's suspension of its proactive recommendation of HPV vaccination. The prolonged suspension and indecision of leadership gave space to the highly networked and proactive parents' group driving an anti-HPV vaccination campaign that was embedding mainstream and social media, paralyzing politicians, and frustrating health professionals. As one Japanese health official told me, "we just do not know how to handle all the emotion."

***

The challenge is that the girls' symptoms are very real. The focus on delinking the symptoms from the vaccine by the medical and scientific community feels like a denial of the girls' experience and pain and further fuels the alienation and anger felt by those affected, including their mothers or others caring for them.

This phenomenon is not unique to Japan, but the Japanese government is the only one to have suspended its proactive recommendation of the vaccine for more than 6 years, garnering applause from vaccine-critical groups[9] while the international scientific community looks on with dismay.

The Japan HPV vaccine story has traveled the world, being featured on vaccine-questioning websites and in films and YouTube videos such as "Sacrificial Virgins" and "The Vitamin Movie," which includes an interview with a Japanese doctor talking about the healing effect of mega doses of vitamin C to treat the persistent shaking and twitches experienced by a group of Japanese girls after HPV vaccination.[10]

The Japan experience and the parent association sparked a number of other associations with similar grievances, including in Spain (Association of Affected People Due to the HPV Vaccine), the United Kingdom (Association of HPV Vaccine Injured Daughters), Ireland (Reactions and Effects of Gardasil Resulting in Extreme Trauma [REGRET]), and Colombia (the Rebuilding Hope Association for HPV Vaccine Victims). The movement went global, enabled by social media networks to not only share information, but also to serve as organizational platforms.

In 2016, the Government of Armenia submitted a proposal to the Global Alliance for Vaccines and Immunization (GAVI) to support a new HPV vaccine program. In the proposal they already anticipated the challenges they expected to face and wrote a concise summary of all the reasons:

> We anticipate that the main impediment in achieving high coverage with HPV vaccine in Armenia will be vaccine safety concerns among the teenage girls, their parents, medical worker and the public in general. . . . Since 2009 only three middle-income countries have introduced HPV vaccine: Romania, The former Yugoslav Republic of Macedonia (MKD), and Kazakhstan. . . . Rumors about negative effects of vaccination on teenage girls' health and scepticism about benefits of HPV vaccination flooded the Internet and social media. As a result, the Ministry of Health of Romania had to cancel HPV vaccination and destroy the vaccine that it had procured. In MKD the HPV vaccine coverage was much lower than coverage for other teenage

vaccines. In Kazakhstan HPV vaccine caused clusters of anxiety-related adverse events following immunization which later transformed into widespread psychogenic reactions that created very negative publicity. As a result, The Ministry of Health of Kazakhstan had to cancel its HPV vaccination program and destroy its vaccine. Recently Denmark and Ireland, high income countries of our region, had similar clusters of anxiety-related AEFIs that negatively affected previously successful HPV vaccination programs. In Denmark the HPV coverage dropped from 86% to 15% within one year. The cluster of anxiety related AEFIs were reported in Japan and lead to suspension of HPV vaccination in this country. The information about vaccine safety events in Kazakhstan, Denmark, and Japan has been broadly disseminated through the Internet, mass media, and social media in all countries of the Region.[11]

Although Armenia has one of the better childhood immunization programs, they knew the HPV vaccine would bring challenges. They were right. Although Armenia was funded and HPV vaccination was offered in 2017, few wanted it for all the reasons they feared. Between December 2 and July 2018, slightly less than 5% of the girls who were offered the vaccine accepted it.

Episodes similar to the Colombia outbreak following HPV vaccination have occurred in the context of a number of different vaccination programs and are not unique to the HPV vaccine. Between 1992 and 2017, diagnoses of MPI following vaccination have occurred around the world—from Australia to Chad,[12] China, Iran, Italy, India, Jordan, Korea,[13] and the United States, to name a few—and have occurred in reaction to a wide variety of vaccines, from those preventing cholera, diphtheria, tetanus, hepatitis B, meningitis, and tetanus, to H1N1 and HPV.[14] In all cases, groups have experienced a range of similar symptoms that were not found to have any link to the specific vaccine, but instead were deemed to be more closely linked to vaccine anxiety, rumors, or other background stresses that fueled the viral spread of emotions and consequent physical symptoms. In each case, the mass reactions—many of which affected school children vaccinated in groups—had dramatic symptoms that further heightened any small anxieties or concerns that the children may have had. In some cases, the children fainted one after the other, like dominoes. They trembled, felt faint, and some experienced convulsions—frightening for anyone to see and enough to provoke panic.

These symptoms are very real, including pain, and can persist for months and years. Hearing that your symptoms are psychological is rarely welcome or even accepted. In 1998, in Amman, Jordan, a tetanus-diphtheria vaccination program was launched in schools. Nearly 20,000 children were vaccinated during the month of September, but on the morning of September 29, 80 children went to the hospital claiming a range of symptoms: fever, headache, aches, nausea, dizziness, and fainting. By the end of the next day, 122 were admitted to the hospital, and the news went viral through local media. The Ministry of Health conducted a survey in all the schools to assess the scope of the reactions, and they found that more than 800 children had reported symptoms, although all of their laboratory tests were normal. Although some of the minor reactions were attributed to the vaccination, the overall investigation concluded MPI. The report pointed not only to vaccine fears—spread through rumors and amplified by the media—but to a background of distrust and discontent with the government. The vaccine saga occurred on the heels of public debates around suspected contamination of the public water supply. The mass illness was not just about the vaccine anxiety: there was deeper fertile ground—deeper distrust from outside the vaccination program that gave ferment to the vaccine anxieties and mass reaction.[15]

A few years earlier, in a rural village in Iran, a tetanus vaccination program was launched in a local school. Four days after the first 26 girls were immunized, one of them fainted and had tremors, headaches, and what was diagnosed as pseudoseizures. Suspecting links to the vaccine, she was examined and was found to have a history of depression and had experienced similar symptoms at other times before the vaccination. Nonetheless, in the following days, nine other girls who had been vaccinated also started having similar symptoms. In these cases, there was no previous history of depression. Without a clear explanation, the outbreak was explained as a psychogenic reaction, likely triggered by the first girl's reactions. For those affected, though, the diagnosis was not comforting. Rumors went viral through the village that the real story was that vaccine had caused a "brain disease,"[16] sparking angst and distrust about the vaccination program. Concerns and fears lingered long after the vaccine reactions.

***

The contagion of emotions and physical symptoms prompted by fear, anxieties, and stress has been studied for decades. During the 20th century these types of symptoms were more commonly associated with concerns about air, food, and water quality.[17] Mass outbreaks of illness are particularly well-documented around chemical incidents where anxiety is high and even an unusual odor can trigger the suggestion of being poisoned, provoking nausea, fainting, tics, and other neurological symptoms—physical symptoms that can spread like wildfire across populations, albeit not actually caused by a toxic substance.

In the summer of 1999, a group of school children in Belgium[18] complained of headache, nausea, breathing problems, dizziness, and trembling. The one thing they all had in common was having drunk Coca-Cola. They were sent to the hospital where multiple lab tests were run, but the tests were all normal. In the following days, children in multiple schools also complained of similar symptoms, complaining of a funny smell in the Coca-Cola. Rumors and anxiety spread through the general population and beyond Belgium. Despite no confirmed link between the Coca-Cola drinks and the illness, Belgium, France, and Spain banned the sale of Coca-Cola and other soft drinks.

The Coca-Cola scare was set against a background of public distrust in Belgium stemming from what became known as the "dioxin crisis." Earlier in the same year as the Coca-Cola events, the public learned of animal feed contamination, with implications for the public food supply. The government had not disclosed this information for months, trying to avert panic but instead creating distrust and adding credibility to the possibility of things going wrong. In addition to the physical distress and anxiety caused by the event, the overall incident cost the Coca-Cola company more than US$100 million.[19] If a risk or rumor is believable enough, it can have a powerful impact on individual as well as collective behavior, with all its resulting human as well as financial costs.

Social media is believed to be also changing the pattern of the mass outbreaks of psychosomatic illness. In 2011, a group of girls developed facial tics and involuntary twitching at Le Roy High School in New York,[20] symptoms which some suspected, like the Coca-Cola incident, were due to a toxic substance, perhaps from a historic chemical spill.[21] Physicians wondered if the bizarre movements were spread by YouTube videos that the girls were posting. As soon as media coverage stopped, they began to recover. One of the neurologists who treated some of the girls commented "It's remarkable to see how one individual posts something, and then the next person who posts something . . . not only are the movements bizarre and not consistent with known movement disorders, but it's the same kind of movements. This mimicry goes on with Facebook or YouTube exposure. This is the modern way that symptomatology could be spread."[22]

Social media also seems to have changed the pattern of these outbreaks. Historically, there have been two types of symptoms. The first is triggered by extreme, sudden stress within a close-knit group and causes symptoms such as dizziness, headaches, and fainting, with those affected generally recovering within 24 hours. A second type arises from longer term anxieties, and the symptoms include shaking, twitching, walking difficulties, and sometimes even uncontrollable laughing. These can last for weeks or months. By sharing videos of these symptoms through social media, there is a new mix of these symptoms occurring, and they are appearing in different locations other than those in which they have historically occurred.[23]

As MPI expert Bartholomew and his colleagues write, "We may be witnessing a milestone in the history of MPI where the primary agent of spread will be the Internet and social media networks. . . . It is likely, as indeed is already happening, that their illnesses will now become symbolic of wider issues."[24]

In 2014, a team of researchers inside Facebook conducted an experiment to understand whether emotional contagion can occur without face-to-face interaction between people. The researchers manipulated the emotional content found in their News Feed and their results confirmed that "Emotional states can be transferred to others via emotional contagion, leading people to experience the same emotions *without their awareness.*" More importantly, they confirmed that these emotions can be evoked online, without face-to face interaction.

> In an experiment with people who use Facebook, we test whether emotional contagion occurs outside of in-person interaction between individuals by reducing the amount of emotional content in the News Feed. When positive expressions were reduced, people produced fewer positive posts and more negative posts; when negative expressions were reduced, the opposite pattern occurred. These results indicate that emotions expressed by others on Facebook influence our own emotions, constituting experimental evidence for massive-scale contagion via social networks . . . a form of emotional contagion.[25]

Episodes of what has been characterized as MPI have tied the hands of high-ranking officials and triggered fear across populations. The panic caused by a hypothetical link between MPI symptoms and HPV vaccine is responsible for dramatic drops in HPV vaccination rates in Colombia, Denmark, and Japan. Although these types of events are not new, the newer landscape of social media has fueled the spread and impact of these outbreaks in unprecedented and far less predictable patterns.

***

The viral spread of emotions can allow certain perceptions or beliefs to travel, evolve, and persist, but this spread can also have dramatic impacts on individual and group behavior. Those exposed to these emotions can also have psychologically triggered physical reactions characterized as psychogenic illness or as MPI when spreading across groups.

This emotional contagion can also have very different outcomes, provoking groups of individuals to have physical, albeit psychologically driven, adverse reactions to vaccination. These types of reactions have played out following different vaccinations, but they have been particularly prevalent among young girls, often in school groups, following HPV vaccination.[26] Given the stigma attached to a psychological illness, and the anger of publics when health officials claim that vaccine reaction are psychological, the World Health Organization (WHO) has convened a group to consider rethinking the name given to such reactions. Initially, the term "anxiety reactions" was explored as a possible, less stigmatized characterization of psychologically triggered reactions to vaccination that manifest as physical symptoms—fainting, trembling, mobility issues, eating disorders. More recent discussions concluded that "anxiety" did not cover the scope of reported reactions to vaccines, and the WHO renamed the syndrome *immunization stress related response* and described it as being provoked by "a combination of biological factors occurring within an individual combined with his or her own psychological strengths and vulnerabilities within a particular social context (the biopsychosocial context)."[27] In short, it's complicated, and while a number of these symptoms may be de-linked from the vaccine, they *are* related to the vaccination experience.

[7]

THE POWER OF BELIEF

Ideas, sentiments, emotions, and beliefs possess in crowds a contagious power as intense as that of microbes.

—Gustave Le Bon, *The Crowd*

As I sat in the green room waiting to be called into the popular BBC Victoria Derbyshire TV talk show, I watched a young girl sitting on a sofa on the other side of the room. She was reaching to pick up a paint brush on the coffee table filled with paint tubes and white paper. My eye caught something shining as she turned, and I realized she had a bionic arm—actually two bionic arms. A young teenager with curly blond hair, big eyes, and Wonder Woman arms. In the background, 13-year-old Tilly appeared on the TV screen in the waiting room. It was a trailer for the upcoming program showing a short clip of Tilly putting on make-up with her new digits. Tilly was the next visitor on the talk show, ready to proudly show her new prosthetic arms as her own arms had been lost to meningitis as an infant. In the 10 minutes we sat in the green room together, I watched her determination as she reached for the thin paint brush with her new bionic fingers, the first try slipping through the near-human robotic clutching. She had a glow in her smile, an enthusiasm for her new abilities. I watched as she got up to try to lift the paint brush from a higher surface in the room. She limped slightly, but carried her small frame with grace, led by the eagerness of her new shiny friends, left and right.

When I was called into the TV studio, I thought of Tilly and the life challenges that an infectious disease left her with. It gave me strength to confront what I expected to be a contentious debate between a pro-vaccine mom and a vaccine refuser willing to put her children at risk of potentially disabling infectious diseases because she had stronger beliefs in a "natural" life, free of chemicals, free of vaccines. I walked around the cameras to sit next to the presenter, the two mothers projected on large screens, video-linked from different parts of the country. The older mother, Jo, whose daughter was severely disabled by measles infection, was at home, and told the story of her daughter's disabling condition caused by measles. The younger activist mother, Lottie, with her infant strapped kangaroo-style against her breast, adamantly denied the existence of a robust safety system for vaccines. She refused vaccines for two of her three children after the first one didn't feel well after a vaccination. The two mothers captured the demographics of vaccine skepticism. Social media-savvy millennials regularly feature in surveys as being the more vaccine-skeptical age group, eager to find their own evidence, make their own choices.

After Lottie's perspective was introduced, the presenter turned to ask her why she was ignoring the consensus of leading medical experts. Dismissing the suggestion that she was ignoring experts, Lottie quickly flipped the question upside down. In her eyes the point was that young mothers felt *they* were the ones being ignored. It was the health experts who were not listening to parents, not the other way around. "I think it is really important that we have this discussion. Parents are not having this discussion. We are routinely shut down from having this discussion. There are hundreds of thousands of children who are injured or damaged by vaccines whom nobody listens to. This is why we have groups such as Arnica, who then have regional groups, some of whom are closed but majority are open, in order to be able to discuss things like this with other parents to try to get to the bottom of what's happened to our children."

The sentiment of feeling "shut down" from having a conversation about vaccine risks comes up again and again. It is a strong thread running through the arguments among vaccine-reluctant mothers who feel that they aren't—or weren't—vaccine skeptical until they felt their questions were being dismissed, their views being put down, which only fueled their suspicions of risks and of having the truth withheld. Meanwhile, many have sought out their own answers, come to their own conclusions, and are not willing to budge.

I left the studio and searched for the Arnica parents group on my phone. The mission statement read, "Arnica is a support group for parents, led by parents," which sounded reasonable. "We believe in a holistic approach to health and recognize a grass roots need for debate and practice, especially in this current climate where nutritional supplements, organic food, and homeopathy are under threat." I was a bit surprised by this part, having the impression that homeopathy and organic food had a growing following rather than being under threat, but it is the perception that matters and affects decisions.

Further down the mission statement, it claimed a neutral stance, "We are a non-profit making group and do not advocate one way to health, although we prefer to use alternatives to allopathic medicine where possible for general health. For example, using nutrition and herbs in place of cold medicines, trying cuddles and homeopathy before Calpol[1] and antibiotics, and supporting natural immunity in place of vaccines." The mission statement seemed to have a clear position about vaccines, although they did add "where possible," which at least reflected some openness for other choices.

"Ultimately, we believe that the non-vaccinated child is potentially healthier than the vaccinated child. . . . Our long-term aim is to encourage the sharing of health records from non-vaccinated children and compare them to vaccinated children." They were not wrong in the principle of wanting to compare outcomes of vaccinated and non-vaccinated children—the principle of randomized controlled trials—but it seemed that they were not aware of the years of controlled trials comparing vaccinated and non-vaccinated children conducted long before any vaccine is ever made available to the public.

The Arnica Group is one of many that strongly believe that Mother Nature is powerful enough to ward off diseases, with part of their healthy lifestyle including raising your children "vaccine-free." For some, the choice of not vaccinating gives an impression of not taking risks and that somehow letting nature take its course is more forgivable than the intentional act of vaccinating. For some, but not for all.

The growing trend toward alternative health beliefs—from naturopathy to homeopathy—is becoming part of an overall lifestyle choice that includes organic, anti-GMO (genetically modified organism) and chemical-free foods, paleo diets, fluoride-free water, home births, natural "rhythm" birth control methods over contraceptive pills, and raising children "vaccine-free." While many aspects of a more natural lifestyle are reasonable, some are less effective or even less safe than others when it comes to disease prevention. Some opt for measles and chickenpox parties as a more "natural" way to build immunity, having their children interact with infected children and acquire natural immunity through contracting the disease. One Facebook page offered to "Find a Pox Party Near You" while another sold chickenpox-licked lollipops sent through the mail. A Nashville TV station spotted the woman's posts, in which she also offered to ship spit and cotton swabs, all for a mere $50, payable through PayPal. The woman, Wendy Werkit, told WSMV reporter Kimberly Curth that she had shipped lollipops that had been sucked on by her children, "so that other peoples' kids can get chickenpox."[2] In the case of the chickenpox lollipops marketing, Facebook deleted the page promoting the pops after judging it as being illegal, falling under the same law that prohibits the mailing of any contagious agent, whether anthrax or chickenpox.

The confidence of those promoting alternative approaches is striking, "We, as parents, know what we're doing. Healthy kids don't die from chicken pox, and our children are healthy, generally with extremely strong immune systems."[3]

One rabbi reflected on a measles outbreak in London's Jewish Orthodox community, "the perception (is) that measles is a 'healthy illness.' It's not seen as a great danger to health." He is not alone. Half way around the world in Australia, an impassioned mother wrote a children's book called *Melanie's Marvellous Measles* encouraging children to embrace measles as "natural." The cover is a colorful spring day with lush green grass, bushes of white and purple flowers, Melanie dressed in pink running with her arms outstretches toward a large blue butterfly, and a face of glee and happiness, embracing nature.

The back cover tells the author's story and point of view, "I have experienced many times when my children's vaccinated peers succumb to the childhood diseases they were vaccinated against. Surprisingly, there were times when my unvaccinated children were blamed for their peer's sickness. Something which is just not possible when they didn't have the diseases at all." But the author misses the point of those who point to her unvaccinated child as contributing to the spread of measles. She is correct to say that her child, if not infected with measles, could not personally spread it to someone else. What unvaccinated children create, particularly when clustered in groups, is a hole in the community protection: in other words a path for the measles to travel through, not necessarily making them sick, but allowing others to become sick. Those who are vaccinated contribute to stopping the spread of the virus. The vaccination is enough to stimulate natural antibodies without making a child sick with measles and its consequent risk of complications.

In one article in the *Financial Times* about beliefs like those of the author of *Melanie's Marvellous Measles,* correspondent Tim Harford asks the question "why do such ideas endure?" He argues that it is not because people "believe anything," because many don't believe some of the things they *should* believe. On the contrary, "the problem is not that nobody cares," he writes. "It is that people care so passionately that they will go to great lengths to dismiss contrary evidence. The scepticism isn't lazy; it is energetic."[4]

One Canadian TV comedy program, "The Beaverton," tried to bring some humor to the tension between parents opting for nature and doctors frustrated in their efforts to encourage them to vaccinate. Standing in front of a glass-doored clinic with a sign board promoting "Free Flu Shots," the presenter introduces the program, "Canada's vaccination rates are on the decline. Despite overwhelming evidence that proves they are safe and effective, their reputation has been harmed by the three D's—Debunked studies, Disgraced former doctors and D-list actors. But now doctors have found a way to convince sceptics to trust vaccines—disguising them as naturopathic treatments!"

In the background, a white-coated doctor walks out of the clinic and hangs another sign over the "Free Flu Shot" board. This one says "Free-Range Turmeric Shots" with a large "Fair Trade" mark stamped below.

The image cuts to the doctor back at her desk talking with the TV presenter. "People will put *anything* in their body if they think it is natural. So, rather than tell people I am giving their kid the mumps vaccine, I just say it's apple cider vinegar! Somehow that's better."

Background images come onto the screen of pamphlets on bee venom, jade eggs, and bras causing breast cancer.

"Doctors call it the 'Goop effect,' continues the presenter, alluding to Gwyneth Paltrow's holistic health promotion. "The idea that natural means safe and endorsed by a celebrity means natural. And now doctors are co-opting it to give all their patients all the benefits of science, without the 'sciency' part that they hate so much." This comes against a background image of the doctor posting a new sign on her door saying "Wellness Buddy," covering the old "Doctor's Office" label. She goes into her office to put on a red floral spa robe instead of white coat and then tacks a "Chakkra System" poster on her wall featuring an Indian cross-legged yogi.

The camera turns back to the doctor. "Once I realized that many patients are convinced that all doctors are in the pocket of 'Big Herd Immunity,' I had a choice to make. Cite peer reviewed studies on vaccinations *or* just tell them it is a shot of good old fashioned 'Healing Juice.'" She lifts a vaccine vial and presses on a new "Healing Juice" label.

"So, you're lying?" the show's presenter asks the Doctor.

"Sure, but least now I can actually treat my patient."

"So," wraps up the presenter, "while the granolification of Canada's health care system may worry those who prefer science-based medicine, it has finally given many parents what they always wanted. A chance to feel smarter than their doctors."

Funny? Probably not for those who are devotees of organic over scientific treatments, but it is a poignant capturing of two polarized worlds, not unlike my experience sitting between Lottie and Jo on the morning talk show.

There is something powerful, almost religiously compelling for some, when it comes to trust in nature. When disease happens "naturally" it is somehow more acceptable and begets less guilt than would any potential side effects from a vaccine. Psychologists call it the "omission bias," where choosing *not* to take an action, such as not getting a vaccination and instead letting nature take its course, feels like a lesser risk with less culpability, even when that action would ultimately reduce a greater risk.

THE FLUIDITY OF RELIGIOUS BELIEFS

The use of religion to either persuade or dissuade publics from vaccination is not uncommon; religion is sometimes used as a guise for other underlying concerns, beliefs, or political stances, or to appeal to the trust networks within a community of shared beliefs. Most religious texts were inscribed well before vaccines existed, and few current religions forbid all vaccines, but instead have issues with specific vaccines or their timing of administration, such as with the age of administration of the HPV vaccine given its association with sexual behavior, or with additives such as the use of fetal tissue in the preparation of some vaccines. Religious reasons for vaccine refusal also vary considerably within religious groups, often depending on an individual religious leader's interpretation of the text or depending on where particular religious groups live and whether they are in the minority or majority, marginalized or supported by government. Those who live as a marginalized or minority group are sometimes less prone to trust the government, particularly when they feel they are not given the same level of services as the rest of the population. This deeper distrust can affect their willingness to participate in a government-driven vaccination program. Some religious groups fear vaccines when they are perceived as being provided by another religious group whose motives they do not trust.

A telling example is one study in Kartoum, Sudan, where the researchers were told, "there is an escalation of religious refusal, for instance; groups such as Ansar Al-Sunna and Wahabia [religious groups] think that vaccines are brought by Jews, for which reason, they refuse all vaccines." While another reported "sometimes they talk about Freemasons and infidel states which bring vaccines."[5]

Divisions within religious groups can also mean different views on vaccination, sometimes with fatal outcomes, as in Pakistan and Nigeria where Muslim, particularly female, polio vaccinators have been killed. These killings were motivated by extremist Muslims who were against not only girls being schooled, but also working in a public role or, even worse, participating in a global vaccination initiative largely funded and driven by Western countries.

Religious leaders have played important roles in both restoring trust in vaccines as well as undermining it. The World Health Organization (WHO) reached out to the Vatican to help rebuild confidence in the tetanus vaccine when the 1995 sterilization rumors circulated in multiple countries. They felt that the Vatican would have more influence in building confidence and trust in the vaccine among its following than any health officials could manage.

A decade later, the WHO reached out to the Organization of Islamic Cooperation to help in overturning the polio vaccination boycott in northern Nigeria that was contributing to the spread of polio locally as well as across multiple countries in Africa. In addition to local rumors that the vaccines could make their children sterile, the polio vaccines were being refused by Muslims who were concerned about the porcine (derived from pork) products in the gelatin used in the oral vaccines. The concern was addressed in a collaborative meeting between the WHO and the Islamic Organization of Medical Scientists who endorsed the use of porcine products.[6] The verdict was that the gelatin had gone through a process that transformed the ingredients of concern to be pure enough for use, and, from a public health perspective, vaccines were allowed in the absence of an alternative, more *halal* option. While this high-level, global agreement helped to mitigate concerns in many countries, local populations still rely on their local imam to give them guidance, some of whom still adamantly believe that porcine products in vaccines are not acceptable for the faithful.

In Malaysia, despite the national Islamic authority endorsing vaccines, the northern state of Kedah had the highest rate of vaccine refusal due to circulating doubts about their halal status. In an interview with Reuters the Malaysian Health Minister S. Subramaniam reported that number of vaccine refusals "more than doubled in the past three years to reach 1,541 in 2015 . . . Our concern is, if it's left uncontrolled, in the long-term we might see a significant effect on the nation as a whole." Already in June 2016, 5 children died of diphtheria due to lack of vaccination.

Among those supporting the vaccine-wary Muslims was Arif Faizal, a proponent and practitioner of alternative medicine in Malaysia. He spoke up for the parents' right to refuse vaccination, but the subtext was that they should have the right to choose alternative medicine—and he had a solution to offer. He was among those who influenced refusing parents, many of whom were all living in Kedah state, reflecting the strong influence of local leadership and tight communities with shared beliefs.[7]

In southern India, similar dynamics evolved when some communities began to resist vaccination for a mix of questions around *halal* compatibility, safety concerns, and fears of sterilization. There, too, a naturopathy guru stepped in to discourage vaccine acceptance. In a Facebook video, Jacob Vadakkanchery, locally known for his anti-vaccine views, pointed to US courts and vaccine safety concerns and suggested that "India gives vaccines which were boycotted in America."[8] He had an alternative approach to offer.

In 2018, Indonesia faced similar resistance seen in Malaysia and southern India. A *fatwa* (religious order) was issued by the Indonesian Ulema Council claiming that the measles, mumps, rubella (MMR) vaccine contained porcine products and was not *halal*, but ambiguously added that it was allowed because there was no available alternative.[9] Despite the *fatwa* which allowed the vaccine, vaccine anxieties and reluctance persisted. And, once again, one of the outspoken advocates of vaccine dissent was a Muslim naturopath, Dewi Hestyawati, promoting "cupping" therapy as an alternative to vaccination.[10]

In some instances, the beliefs that drive vaccine reluctance or refusal are less about resistance to vaccination and more about specific ingredients. Vaccines that involve the use of aborted fetal tissue are rejected by some religious groups who are opposed to abortion, while others will not accept the use of porcine products in the gelatin used in some oral vaccine capsules or for nasal vaccines because it is derived from pork.[11]

Vaccine decisions are rarely determined by a single belief, but rather from an interweaving of different strands of values and beliefs—whether religious, philosophical, or naturopathic. This web of beliefs helps to rationalize and navigate uncertainties, fears, and anxieties around vaccines, particularly when the trust relationship with those providing the vaccines is tenuous.

WHEN BELIEFS FUEL VIOLENCE

In 2007, 24,000 children were not vaccinated in Pakistan's North West Frontier. Parents distrusted the foreign-led polio vaccination initiative, and rumored risks of sterilization were stoked by extreme religious clerics using loudspeakers in mosques as well as preaching on radio stations and spreading misinformation about the vaccines. They were motivated not only by their religiosity, but also by anger. In Swat Valley, a militant cleric had lost his brother in an attack on an Islamic school, and he used the radio to express his anger, also undermining the polio vaccination campaign as representative of a government initiative. In the Swat area, 4,000 children did not get vaccinated.[12]

In Bajaur, along the Afghan border, the United States had bombed a house trying to kill one of al-Qaida's leaders, thus angering extremists and further fueling their resistance toward polio vaccination campaigns. In consequence, 2,000 children in the Bajaur area were not vaccinated. Worse, the head of the Bajaur government vaccination campaign was assassinated by militants.

Increased drone strikes by the United States in the same area of Northwest Pakistan escalated tensions between insurgents and the polio vaccination effort. The Taliban commander in the drone-affected area called a ban on polio vaccination in North Waziristan until the drones stopped. More than 160,000 children were blocked from getting their vaccination.[13]

Suspicions and distrust of government and international initiatives only became more entrenched and made credible by the US CIA initiative in Pakistan in 2011. In an effort to verify the hiding place of Osama bin Laden, the CIA chose a fake hepatitis vaccination campaign as a cover for a doctor to enter the suspected hiding place of bin Laden and confirm his presence. The timing came at a fragile moment in the polio eradication efforts in Pakistan, one of the last countries in the world harboring the polio virus. Polio eradication depends on door-to-door vaccination to ensure that every child is vaccinated. The sham door-to-door vaccination brought to bin Laden's door did not help the already waning confidence and trust in these repeated door-to-door polio campaigns.

When news of the CIA fake vaccination campaign broke in *The Guardian* (UK) in 2011, it shook the immunization and public health world. Anxieties and distrust about the polio vaccine and its Western providers were already rampant in some communities, with rumors spreading that the vaccines were sterilizing Muslims in retaliation for 9/11, alongside suspicions about CIA links with the polio eradication campaign.

Aside from the public's distrust and heightened suspicion instilled by the CIA fake immunization deception, the episode further fueled the militants' resistance to the polio vaccination campaign, heightening and reinforcing their suspicion of underlying US motives.

Between December 17 and 19, 2012, nine polio workers were killed. Four were killed in northwest Pakistan, and five were shot and killed in Karachi at the other end of the country. In the same month, across the border, a polio worker in Afghanistan was murdered. Anisa was a young woman in her early 20s, on her way to her first day of work as a polio vaccinator,[14] having been warned by threatening messages not to leave home.

On January 29, 2013, a policeman was killed. He was meant to be protecting polio workers who were trying to continue their work despite the risks. On January 31, two more polio workers were killed.

Seeming to mimic the Pakistan attacks, in February 2013, nine polio workers were murdered in Kano State, Nigeria, home of the polio vaccination boycott a decade earlier.[15] The previous October, two security guards had also been killed in Nigeria while working to protect the vaccinators. This had become not a war on polio, but a war on the polio program.

The violence was not only directed toward polio workers and the polio initiative; it was part of a broader landscape of militancy, local and global politics, and a clash of values and religions. Anisa was killed 2 months after a gunman shot the now celebrated Malala Yousafzai because she had stood up for girls' education. In January 2013, a month before the nine polio workers were killed, militants bombed a Shia Muslim minority mosque, killing 120 people, and, in September 2013, more than 80 people were killed in a church in Peshawar because they were Christian. In 2014, a school in Peshawar was targeted and 141 were killed. These attacks were against freedom—freedom to choose to go to school, to go to church, or to give or receive a polio vaccine.

On March 6, 2013, a health center was bombed in the Khyber Agency, northwest of Peshawar, Pakistan. One polio worker inside the center was injured, and others might have been injured or killed had the bomb exploded when the polio workers were scheduled to meet a little later that morning. In response, three political administration officials and five tribal police officers were arrested for negligence. But no one has been arrested for the actual killings.

On March 7, 2013, three polio vaccinators working together were assaulted and threatened with death if they attempted to vaccinate children in that area. The assault took place about 30 kilometers from the bombed health center. No one was arrested for the assault.

In October 2013, the news of two more polio-related killings in Pakistan—this time a policeman and a member of a peace group helping to deliver polio vaccination supplies—was seen as a message to the polio eradication campaign. With the news of the CIA ploy using a fake hepatitis vaccination initiative to confirm the location of Osama bin Laden, militants were convinced that the polio workers were engaged in US surveillance activity to guide drone attacks. Hence, the US political decision to use vaccination as a ploy to find bin Laden trumped a global health priority in the context of what has been perceived as more important global security concerns, but not without trust-breaking consequences.[16] Actions such as the CIA hoax vaccination give credence to conspiracy theorists, making rumors more credible and serving as a global "told you so" by those already suspicious of state or international interventions.

In January 2013, the deans of 12 public health schools across the United States sent a letter to President Obama, appealing to him to never again allow covert action to be embedded in a public health effort.

In September Save the Children was forced by the Government of Pakistan (GoP) to withdraw all foreign national staff. This action was apparently the result of CIA having used the cover of a fictional vaccination campaign to gather information about the whereabouts of Osama Bin Laden. In fact, Save the Children never employed the Pakistani physician serving the CIA, yet in the eyes of the GoP he was associated with the organization. This past month, eight or more United Nations health workers who were vaccinating Pakistani children against polio were gunned down in unforgivable acts of terrorism. While political and security agendas may by necessity induce collateral damage, we as an open society set boundaries on these damages, and we believe this sham vaccination campaign exceeded those boundaries.[17]

In May 2014, the deans received a reply. The Director of the CIA confirmed that there would be no further operational use of vaccine programs, including vaccinators, nor would they "seek to identify or exploit DNA or genetic material" (as they had attempted with Bin Laden). A little too late.

In August 2014, the WHO announced that two children were found paralyzed by polio harbored behind Boko Haram militants in inaccessible Borno State.[18] This occurred 2 years after what many had hoped to be the last case of polio not only in Nigeria but in all of Africa. Had the local health officials and global health community been able to interrupt the Nigeria boycott a decade earlier instead of dismissing early rumors and believing they would somehow go away, perhaps the world might have eradicated polio by now. Instead, conflict, insecurity, and overt violence against polio workers have plagued the eradication efforts, and polio returned to Nigeria after a hopeful few years when it seemed have been eliminated.

13 January 2016, Attempts to eradicate poliomyelitis in Pakistan, one of the last refuges of the crippling disease, received a setback on January 13 (2016) after a bomb blast near the main polio centre in Quetta, capital of Balochistan province, left 13 policemen and two other people dead.[19]

In January 2018, Sakina Bibi, 38, and her daughter, Rizwana, 16, were giving drops to children when two gunmen on a motorcycle opened fire, killing both in the southwestern city of Quetta. On April 24, 2019, a gunmen shot and killed a police officer guarding a polio immunization team in northern Pakistan.[20] And two more polio workers were killed.

These situations demonstrate the power of belief-driven emotions in unleashing violence and sparked by a vaccination campaign that touched a religious and political nerve. While the situation in Pakistan has its own unique set of challenges for polio eradication, the fundamental issue of restricted freedom there is not unlike the biggest challenge facing polio eradication in Northern Nigeria. There, Islamic militants—namely Boko Haram—are threatening the daily lives and freedoms of not just polio workers, but also of many others. Polio vaccination attacks are just one of many attacks on freedoms, on association with the Western world, and on beliefs that are not consistent with those of the militants.

In the face of persisting violence around the polio vaccination effort, the International Monitoring Board of the Polio Eradication Initiative asked the question "are the right people in the right jobs? Traditionally, the Program's strengths have lain with technical and epidemiological disease control interventions and activities, but this is different."[21]

The story had only become more complex, with many of the challenges extending beyond the scope of the global polio program. With the killing of polio workers and fears around vaccinations, the virus began spreading rapidly. Security analysts pointed to jihadists as a new risk, carrying polio from Pakistan to other countries on their trail. The stream of jihadists from Pakistan to Syria increased in early 2012. By December, two children with the tell-tale paralysis of polio were identified in Syria's eastern province of Dayr az Zawr, which was under the control of Islamist rebel factions. Syria had not seen a case of polio for a decade.

By November 2013, the polio had spread, paralyzing 36 children across Syria. By March 2014, following the trail of jihadists, new polio cases broke out in Iraq.[22] Genetic sequencing by the US Centers for Disease Control and Prevention (CDC) identified the strain as coming from Pakistan.[23]

The polio eradication effort had become a stage for acting out other issues, using rumors of sterilization, questioning the motives of the international actors, and using violence against vaccinators to disrupt what many had envisioned as being a global health good.

[8]

PANDEMICS AND PUBLICS

In 1918, the world faced the devastating H1N1 influenza pandemic, which sickened 500 million people globally and killed 50 million, with some estimates being closer to 100 million.[1] There was no available vaccine or treatment. There was also far less available information, some unknown and some purposefully suppressed to keep the public focused on World War I. It was the most fatal pandemic since the Black Death of the 14th century. Communication between families and their loved ones heading off to war and news about the spread of the flu was largely through handwritten letters, and that was only when they had an address to send to. Time moved at a different pace, and uncertainty was high. Despite the significant deaths and disabling illness around the world, there was little panic, perhaps due to this very lack of information or because "the flu" is such a common occurrence.

In India, the 1918 influenza pandemic came on the heels of a bubonic plague outbreak that had killed nearly 10 million people by 1921. Rumors around the plague and the extensive disinfecting measures across Mumbai provoked panic, and almost half of the city's 850,000 population fled, contributing to the spread of the disease outside of Mumbai.[2] But while the plague had sparked a contagion of both infection and emotions, the 1918 H1N1 Influenza, which killed nearly 18 million people in India,[3] experienced a very different response. As historian Robert Peckham writes in his introduction to *Empires of Panic*, "where plague provoked a major panic that affected both the colonial regime and the Indian population, sparking rumor, riots, repression, and mass migration from urban centers, the greater and more abrupt mortality of the influenza episode passed without any apparent crisis."[4]

One hundred years later, we are caught in the quagmire of too much rather than too little information. Some of it is lost in translation, some is intentionally manipulated. Which information can we trust? Who can we trust? What is real, what is "fake"? Who is real and who is fiction and designed to fit your profile of "friends"—all those you "trust," although you have never met?

The familiarity of influenza is one of the drivers of complacency around flu vaccination. In the wake of the 2009 worldwide H1N1 "swine flu" pandemic, the World Health Organization (WHO) sounded alarm bells around the potential for widespread deaths, and alarmist news headlines started circulating. In London, initial news headlines alerting the public that "100,000 Londoners to Die of Pig Flu!" calmed a bit in the coming days, but the news still reported warnings of a possible 65,000 swine (H1N1) flu deaths, with many articles evoking memories of the devastating 1918 "Spanish Flu." Despite the sirens, there was little panic among the public, and the global uptake of the H1N1 vaccine was dismal.

In the background, other memories were also circulating of the less distant 1976 swine flu outbreak, which prompted the United States to call for a vaccination campaign that went wrong, with the vaccine showing links to an increased risk of the neurological condition Guillain-Barre syndrome. Although the 2009 vaccine was a newer, improved vaccine, memories lingered.

A Babelian mix of truths, partial truths, and intentional lies has taken a toll on public trust in science. Waning vaccine confidence, skepticism about the safety and even the need for vaccines, and an overall tectonic shift away from trusting "experts" to having more confidence in the opinions and "evidence" shared in stories circulating among neighbors, friends, colleagues, and online social networks speak to a near reversal of the Age of Enlightenment. Three hundred years ago, science was championed as freedom from religious dogma. Today science has become the new dogma. To some, it feels inaccessible, didactic, and impersonal, stripped of the human emotions of daily life.

Instead, personal stories alongside religious and philosophical beliefs are regaining ground, including some retreating to Mother Nature in lieu of scientifically proved health interventions. There is widespread trust in anything natural, tangible, and untampered with by modern man.

While there is an abundance of science and evidence that has demonstrated the value and effectiveness of vaccines, the landscape of publicly available vaccine information is more ambiguous than ever. A confusing mix of scientific evidence, real or perceived risks and rumors, personal or heard experiences together seed a landscape of doubt. It is not merely the ambiguity of facts, though, that is fueling the search for alternative evidence. As epidemiologist Stephen Ledeer rightly points out, "Facts are not rejected because they are seen as being wrong, but because they are seen as being irrelevant."[5] People believe in other approaches, they have different values. There is a burgeoning realm of natural and alternative medicine, as well as philosophical and religious doctrines, promoting ways to keep immune systems strong and vaccine-free. And they have a growing following.

Adult vaccination, in general, has considerably lower acceptance than childhood vaccination. But the low-to-no acceptance of H1N1 vaccines around the world, including among health professionals should be a wake-up call.

The world was lucky that the anticipated fatalities of the 2009 H1N1 pandemic were far less than expected. But if the world responds to the next high-risk pandemic with the same level of vaccine reluctance it did in response to H1N1, we may not be so lucky. It is time to not only understand what went wrong, but to start acting on it to build the public's trust—and the public health community's trustworthiness—before the next pandemic hits.

The WHO became a particular target of outrage at the seemingly exaggerated proclamations of global flu deaths that prompted large-scale government purchases of the H1N1 vaccine,[6] triggering speculation about financial motives and rumors about WHO links to the pharmaceutical industry.[7] France alone spent almost a billion euros on 94 million H1N1 vaccines, but only 5 million of the 65 million population got the vaccine, and it was deemed a "fiasco."[8] News headlines reflected the anger, "H1N1 France: From Vaccine Refusal to Police Riot in Just Seven Days."

One of the striking aspects of the public response was the issue of timing. Danielle Ofri, a medical doctor, wrote a poignant story of the changing sentiments of her patients. They were initially keen to have the not-yet-available vaccine, but, by the time it was available, interest in the vaccine had waned as the pandemic did not seem to be as fatal as anticipated. It seemed to be "just the flu." In reality, it was different. The 2009 H1N1 flu killed adolescents and otherwise healthy adults, unlike the usual trend of infants too young to be vaccinated and others with weaker immune systems being the most likely to succumb to the flu. Dr. Ofri reflected on patient patterns and referred to the "emotional epidemiology" she witnessed alongside the disease epidemiology, pointing to the importance of "treating both (emotions and disease) with equal urgency."[9]

In India, health authorities could not understand why their limited stock of the 2009 H1N1 vaccine was being refused by health workers. Researchers from Greece, Israel, Turkey, and China, were also asking "what went wrong?" Numerous vaccine experts met to try to understand why—in the face of a serious pandemic threat—many people didn't want the vaccine. The conclusion to their final report, aptly titled "Crisis of Public Confidence in Vaccines," was clear. "To not take action now to improve public confidence in vaccines will risk seeing the return of the infectious disease scourges of the past."[10]

The winter of 2017–2018, was a particularly bad season for annual influenza with an estimated 45 million people becoming infected, over 800,000 hospitalized and 61,000 dying in the United States.[11] Yet, despite the severity and number of annual deaths, there is a persisting complacency around a disease that is often talked about as "just the flu." The flu response in the United States was dramatically different, almost indifferent, compared to the excessive panic seen around the feared risks of Ebola during the 2014-2016 West Africa outbreak, even though, in the United States, there were a total of 11 people treated for Ebola and 2 who died. As Sandman lists in his components that define risk perception, this fits the category "Is it familiar or exotic?"

The flu, despite the death tolls it is responsible for, is all too familiar—unless you are a mother who loses a child to the flu. In a premier screening of the 2017 feature film *Unseen Enemy*, investigating contemporary threats of infectious diseases, I sat on the stage next to Gwen and Terry Zwanziger. We had all been interviewed in the film, and we were there to have a discussion with the audience. Gwen and Terry had the most compelling tale.[12] Their 17-year-old daughter Shannon had died of the flu. After a week of "normal" flu, she had been sent home from the doctor to "just rest" and had died in her mother's arms after only 1 week of being ill.

Shannon's parents had never been to New York City and had traveled by train from Minnesota to participate in the panel. This was the first time they would see the film. I was sitting near them in the audience and could feel the emotions and see tears welling in their eyes when Shannon's story came on the screen. It was hard to imagine how painful the experience must have been and how brave they were to come and face a New York audience to talk about their loss.

On stage, the predictable "What did it feel like to watch the film for the first time?" question was posed to them. Unflinchingly, Terry said "it wasn't as difficult as the real thing." They both talked about how important it was for them to tell their story and to alert other parents of the seriousness of flu, even for an otherwise healthy and fit teenager. Gwen talked about having given her daughter the choice of whether she wanted a flu vaccination or not. Her daughter had chosen not to have the vaccine, and Gwen deeply regretted not having tried to convince her otherwise. She herself hadn't realized how serious the risk of not vaccinating really was and that the flu could kill her daughter.

Gwen talked about her Facebook group "Flu Moms," where mothers whose children have died of flu support each other and share their experiences. She said the support group helped tremendously, but the difficult memory lives on. Her mission is to help prevent others from going through what her family went through.

***

There are a growing number of stories of individuals and groups standing up for vaccines, using their personal stories to create a different narrative, including children.

In early 2019, an Ohio teenager, Ethan Lindenberger started a Reddit thread. He went to the "Stupid Questions" page and wrote, "My parents are kind of stupid and don't believe in vaccines. Now that I'm 18, where do I go to get vaccinated? Can I get vaccinated at my age?"

His question made it to the mainstream news, and he ended up speaking in Congress before a full Committee Hearing on "Vaccines Save Lives: What Is Driving Preventable Disease Outbreaks?"[13]

He explained his story in the Reddit post, "As the title explains, my parents think vaccines are some kind of government scheme. It's stupid, and I've had countless arguments over the topic. But, because of their beliefs, I've never been vaccinated for anything, god knows how I'm still alive. But, I'm a senior in high school now with a car, a license, and money of my own. I'd assume that I can get them on my own but I've just never had a conversation with anyone about the subject. I'm also afraid I'd go somewhere that up charges vaccines way more than somewhere just down the street. Any advice would be awesome."

In a new post, he posted: "I have an appointment in a few weeks to get my shots! My mom was especially angry but my dad said because I'm 18 he doesn't care that much. Although my mom's trying to convince me to not do it and saying I don't care about her, I know that this is something I need to do regardless."[14]

Ethan got his vaccinations and has started a newwave of pro-vaccine advocacy, going where the future goes: Online.

In September 2019, Ethan spoke at the World Vaccine Summit hosted by the European Commission in Brussels. As I sat next to him on the speakers' row he seemed a bit nervous, looking around the formal hall that resembles a smaller version of the UN Security Council chamber, with name plates bearing the countries represented. His nervousness faded when he was called to the podium. He had a story to tell and a message to share. He talked about growing up in a household where vaccines were considered scary and with a mother who talked openly about her belief that vaccines cause autism. He talked about his decision to go against his mother and get his vaccinations when he was legally able to at age 18, and he had the conviction to speak up and try to influence those around him who hadn't made a decision yet, convinced that his mother would never change her mind. He stressed the importance of getting the message to his generation, *from* his generation.

But Ethan had another plea and that was about the problem of misinformation and how he felt it needed to be approached differently. "My message in my platform isn't just that vaccines work," he said firmly, "it is about misinformation."

"Misinformation about vaccines can come in many forms," he continued thoughtfully, sounding like a college professor, "and it is not just about the side effects. There are misinformed ideas that there is even a debate around vaccines. That's not true. The debate around vaccines is a lie. That is misinformation in itself. The science has decided vaccines are safe and effective. Legitimizing the idea that there is a debate around vaccines is dangerous, it is a problem in itself.

"And, there are other misinformed ideas, that people who are against vaccines are bad people, that my mom is a malicious person. That is not true. She is a loving mother. If you think about it in this way . . . they [people like her] are doing it for the same reasons that we speak here today. It is about a concern for children's safety. That is why my mother didn't vaccine me. So clarifying that kind of empathy and respect and understanding is really important, instead of demonizing the other side and the misinformed individuals that have fallen into this rabbit hole, you extend them a hand and build bridges.

"This disease of misinformation, it has no cure. My mother will probably never change her views, she will end up living her entire life until her deathbed, believing that vaccines cause autism. But instead of demonizing her and other people and saying they are the problem, we need to find solutions."

That was the message from a teenager. An appeal for kindness, empathy, and understanding.

***

Emotions are rising. While medical and scientific powers somehow expect the old rules and hierarchies to hold their ground, hoping that publics will finally come to their senses and that a few disease outbreaks will motivate them to line up for their vaccinations, new rules of engagement are being decided outside of esteemed institutions. New relationships are being established and new notions of "evidence" taking hold.

Vaccines sit on the cusp of these transformations, embedded in government processes, produced by big business, innovated by scientific discovery, and navigating the wonders as well as the consequences of a digital revolution that has supported and disrupted local and global politics and touched almost every human life on the planet. The vaccine enterprise, from discovery to delivery, cannot escape the turbulence that surrounds it.

While the scientific community ponders how to navigate this new relationship, the public has already moved ahead, doing their own research, finding their own evidence—with Google and social media at their fingertips and growing networks of like-minded people reinforcing their beliefs and anxieties. Already in 2002, only 4 years after Google was launched, Julie Leask and colleagues at the University of Sydney, published a study showing that when "vaccination" was searched across 7 of the most used search engines 43% of the top ten results across all platforms had anti-vaccine content, but for Google the first 10 results were 100% anti-vaccine content.[15]

Today, we are in the paradoxical situation of having better vaccine science and more vaccine safety regulations and processes than ever before, but a doubting public. People are asking whether we really need so many vaccines. Are they safe? Why can't we (the public) choose what we want? What are the real motives behind vaccination? Political gain? Economic gain by governments and the pharmaceutical companies? Who is the state to impose mandates on our freedom of choice and impose on our religious or other beliefs?

One of the challenges is that the health and immunization community has taken so long to take seriously the growing concerns and anxieties of individuals that some of these views have hardened to a point of no return, further nursed by the broader societal and political polarization in which the vaccine debates are situated. The debates around vaccines have become entwined with geopolitical issues, as well as with local political campaigns, religious and other belief-driven identities, celebrity causes, and age-old but newly evolved devotion to Mother Nature. While some people are merely hesitant, yet continue to vaccinate, others are more extreme, joining their anti-vaccine views with other sentiments from environmental (anti-chemical and anti-mercury) groups to those protesting government control, anti-abortion, and even anti-migration—building constituencies well beyond vaccine circles.

What is particularly striking is the deep distrust in the motives— political, business, and research motives—that prompt suspicions and extend beyond national entities to international health bodies. The assumption that populations would accept—and continue to accept—more and more vaccines needs a reality check. As one publication on the history of anti-vaccination movements aptly concludes, "vaccination is unique among de facto mandatory requirements in the modern era, requiring individuals to accept the injection of a medicine or medicinal agent into their bodies, and it has provoked a spirited opposition. This opposition began with the first vaccinations, has not ceased, and probably never will."[16]

Yet, despite these historic and current waves of opposition, vaccines will continue to be a crucial tool to prevent—and potentially eradicate—disabling and fatal diseases. We have created a planet dependent on them.

The global vaccine enterprise needs to reboot because the assumptions that publics around the world will continue to seek and accept increasing numbers of vaccines because they address a public health goal and save lives is just not good enough. The deeper persisting beliefs about basic freedoms, having a voice, and being respected are incontestable. Vaccines need to have meaning in the context of a complex web of emotions, politics, and principles, owned by the public more than ever.

Dr. King's speech when he received the Nobel Peace Prize in 1964, 4 years before his assassination, captured a still persisting challenge.

> Modern man has brought this whole world to an awe-inspiring threshold of the future. He has reached new and astonishing peaks of scientific success. He has produced machines that think and instruments that peer into the unfathomable ranges of interstellar space. . . . This is a dazzling picture of modern man's scientific and technological progress.
>
> Yet, in spite of these spectacular strides in science and technology, and still unlimited ones to come, something basic is missing. There is a sort of poverty of the spirit which stands in

glaring contrast to our scientific and technological abundance. We have learned to fly the air like birds and swim the sea like fish, but we have not learned the simple art of living together.[17]

Immunization has become a profound test of our ability to cooperate. The global spread of viruses punctuates human history, wiping out populations, risking the survival of indigenous populations, and disrupting the productive and social lives of families and communities through disabling disease and death.[18] Vaccines interrupted those patterns of disease, saving millions of lives and, in some cases, saving whole communities, as in Peru in 2005, when the government urgently called for a hepatitis B vaccination campaign not only to save individual lives, but also to prevent an entire indigenous group from slipping into extinction.

The quality of life that most of us enjoy today is dependent on vaccines. In many ways it is one of the biggest worldwide social experiments in collectivism and cooperation in modern times. The challenge is that it depends on a social contract whose fabric is eroding in a broader context of anti-globalization, nationalism, and populism. Vaccines can, as they have in the past, serve as a form of soft diplomacy to keep at least a fundamental level of global cooperation alive and well.

In a thoughtful article reflecting on a post-911 world, and heightened concerns about bio-terrorism, vaccine safety expert Robert Chen recognizes our planetary vaccine-dependency. He also poses the question as to whether the human race will be up to the task of not only sustaining our relationship with vaccines as a way of life, but also adapt as we face each new infectious disease and societal challenge.

"In the larger picture of the struggle of the human species eternal battle against infectious diseases, we are only at the dawning of a new era where immunizations will be needed indefinitely. It remains to be seen whether Homo sapiens will make the necessary adaptations socially and scientifically to sustain and extend the remarkable success of immunizations during this past century."[19]

In the end, I am a patient optimist.

NOTES

Introduction

1. Kulenkampff M, et al. Neurological complications of pertussis inoculation. *Arch Dis Child* 1974;49:46–49.
2. Hussain A, et al. The anti-vaccination movement: A regression in modern medicine. *Cureus* 2018;10(7):e2919.
3. Baker JP. The pertussis vaccine controversy in Great Britain, 1974–1986. *Vaccine* 2003;21:4003–4010.
4. Gangarosa EJ, et al. Impact of anti-vaccine movements on pertussis control: The untold story. *Lancet* 1998;351:356–361.
5. Thousands of Muslim children not being vaccinated against the flu after Kirklees imams reject NHS nasal spray. *Examiner* October 2014. https://www.examiner.co.uk/news/west-yorkshire-news/thousands-muslim-children-not-being-8000201
6. Canadian Bishop under fire for opposing HPV vaccine. Calgary spokeswoman urges Catholic school board to disobey the Bishop Fred Henry. July 2012. http://www.ncregister.com/daily-news/canadian-bishop-under-fire-for-opposing-hpv-vaccine
7. Le Bon G. *The crowd: A study of the popular mind*. New York: Macmillan Co., 1896.
8. http://edition.cnn.com/2015/03/03/asia/pakistan-polio-vaccine-arrests/
9. Karnataka government plans largest vaccination drive, but confusion prevails among schools, parents. https://www.thenewsminute.com/article/

k-taka-govt-plans-largest-vaccination-drive-confusion-prevails-among-schools-parents-55812

10. https://www.dawn.com/news/1475948/women-launch-protest-drive-against-illegal-gas-connections

11. http://www.heartfile.org/blog/860

12. Broniatowski DA, et al. Weaponized health communication: Twitter bots and Russian trolls amplify the vaccine debate. *Am J Public Health* 2018 October 1;108(10):1378–1384.

13. https://www.forbes.com/sites/brucelee/2018/08/25/that-anti-vaccination-message-may-be-from-a-russian-bot-or-troll/#28ab0ca5ff77

14. CDC telebriefing on the national immunization survey, vaccine for children program, and recent measles outbreaks in the US. https://www.cdc.gov/media/releases/2013/t0912_measles-outbreaks-data.html.

15. Knapp RH. A psychology of rumor. *Public Opinion Q* 1944;8(1):22–37.

16. Leach, Melissa, and James Fairhead. 2007. Vaccine anxieties: global science, child health and society. London: Earthscan.

17. Ghinai I, et al. Listening to the rumors: What the northern Nigeria polio vaccine boycott can tell us ten years on. *Global Public Health* 2013;8(10):1138–1150. http://dx.doi.org/10.1080/17441692.2013.859720

18. McDougall, W. *The Group Mind.* Cambridge: Cambridge University Press, 1920.

19. Le Bon, *The crowd,* 17.

20. Salathé M, et al. The dynamics of health behavior sentiments in a large online social network. *EPJ Data Science* 2013;2:4. http://www.epjdatascience.com/content/2/1/4

21. McConnell J. Mass gatherings health Series. *Lancet Infect Dis* 2012 January;(12):8–9.

22. Voss K. On Twitter anti-vaccination sentiments spread more easily than pro-vaccination sentiments. (Interview with Marcel Salathé) *PhysOrg* April 4, 2013. https://phys.org/news/2013-04-twitter-anti-vaccination-sentiments-easily-pro-vaccination.html

23. Rothstein A. Vaccines and their critics, then and now. *New Atlantis* 2015.

24. Armstrong K. Evidence for religious faith: A red herring. In *Evidence,* A. Bell (ed.). Cambridge: Cambridge University Press, 2008: 174–194.

25. Broniatowski DA, et al. Weaponized health communication.

26. TurnerI R, on behalf of the *PLOS Medicine* editors. Measles vaccination: A matter of confidence and commitment. *PLOS Med* 2019;16(3):e1002770.

27. https://www.nytimes.com/2019/09/23/health/anti-vaccination-movement-us.html?searchResultPosition=10

28. Science as an open enterprise. The Royal Society Science Policy Centre report 02/2012, p. 40. https://royalsociety.org/~/media/policy/projects/sape/2012-06-20-saoe.pdf

Chapter 1

1. Allport GW, Postman LJ. The basic psychology of rumor. *Transactions of the New York Academy of Sciences*, 1945;(8):61–81.
2. The Boston Herald. Rumor clinic of World War II. http://www. newenglandhistoricalsociety.com/the-boston-herald-rumor-clinic-of-world-war-ii/
3. Bush GW. State of the union address. January 29, 2002. https://web.archive. org/web/20111011053416/http://millercenter.org/president/speeches/ detail/4540
4. Allport GW, Postman L. An analysis of rumor. *Public Opinion Q* 1946;10(4):501–517.
5. Allport GW, Postman L. *The psychology of rumor*. New York: Henry Holt, 1947.
6. Ibid., 43.
7. Festinger L. A study of rumor: Its origin and spread. *Human Relations* 1948;1:464–485.
8. Hart B. The psychology of rumour. *Proc R Soc Med.* 1916;9(Sect Psych):1–26.
9. Le Bon G. *The crowd: A study of the popular mind*. New York: Macmillan Co., 1896.
10. Prasad J. The psychology of rumor: A study relating to the great Indian earthquake of 1934. *Br J Psychol* 1935;26(1):1–15.
11. DiFonzo N, Bordia P. *Rumor psychology*. Washington, DC: American Psychological Association, 2007.
12. Bordia P, Rosnow RL. Rumor rest stops on the information highway: A naturalistic study of transmission patterns in a computer-mediated rumor chain. *Human Comm Res* 1995;25:163–179.
13. CDC. Epidemiologic notes and reports investigation of a smallpox rumor. *MMRW* 1985;34(23):343–344. https://www.cdc.gov/mmwr/preview/ mmwrhtml/00000557.htm
14. https://apps.who.int/iris/bitstream/handle/10665/155529/WHA33_R4_ eng.pdf;sequence=1
15. WHO. Epidemic intelligence: systematic event detection. https://www.who. int/csr/alertresponse/epidemicintelligence/en/
16. Grein TW, et al. Rumors of disease in the global village: Outbreak verification. *Emerg Infect Dis* 2000;6(2):97–102.
17. Saman G, et al. Rumor surveillance and avian influenza H5N1. *Emerg Infect Dis* 2005;11(3):463–466.
18. Kummervold PE, et al. Controversial Ebola vaccine trials in Ghana: A thematic analysis of critiques and rebuttals in digital news. *BMC Public Health* 2017;17:642.
19. Nerghes A, Kerkhof P, Hellsten L. Early public responses to the Zika-virus on YouTube: Prevalence of and differences between conspiracy theory and

informational videos. Proceedings of 10th ACM Conference on Web Science, Amsterdam, Netherlands, May 27–30, 2018 (WebSci '18), 8 pages. https://doi.org/10.1145/3201064.3201086

20. ScienceBlogs. Zika virus and microcephaly: Anti-vaccine warriors say it's vaccines that did it! https://scienceblogs.com/insolence/2016/02/11/zika-virus-and-microcephaly-antivaccine-warriors-say-its-vaccines-that-did-it

21. Statnews. Zika virus, not vaccine or insecticide, linked to birth defects in Brazil. https://www.statnews.com/2017/12/13/zika-microcephaly-vaccine-insecticide/

22. de Araújo TVB, et al. Association between microcephaly, Zika virus infection, and other risk factors in Brazil. *Lancet Infect Dis* 2018;18:328–336.

23. https://www.pbs.org/wgbh/frontline/article/as-brazil-confronts-zika-vaccine-rumors-shape-perceptions/

24. http://www.annenbergpublicpolicycenter.org/zika-survey-some-incorrectly-link-pesticide-vaccines-to-birth-defect/

25. https://blogs.wsj.com/indiarealtime/2016/02/23/tatas-zica-car-gets-a-new-name-after-virus-outbreak/

26. Gahr P, et al. An outbreak of measles in an undervaccinated community. *Pediatrics* 2014;134(1):e220–8. doi: 10.1542/peds.2013-4260

27. http://www.startribune.com/anti-vaccine-doctor-meets-with-somalis/118547569/

28. Aziz F, Miles SH. Measles, autism and vaccination in the Minnesota Somali community. https://www.mnmed.org/getattachment/news-and-publications/mn-medicine-magazine/Past-Issues/Past-Issues-2018/Jan-Feb-2018/Commentary-Aziz-180102.pdf.aspx?lang=en-US

29. Jama A, Ali M, Lindstrand A, Butler R, Kulane A. Perspectives on the measles, mumps and rubella vaccination among Somali mothers in Stockholm. *Int J Environ Res Public Health* 2018;15:2428. doi:10.3390/ijerph15112428

30. Public Health Agency of Sweden. Barriers and motivating factors to MMR vaccination in communities with low coverage in Sweden Implementation of the WHO's Tailoring Immunization Programmes (TIP) method (2015). https://www.folkhalsomyndigheten.se/contentassets/5db4b41a40f94e98b0e1d0d4a596bae8/barriers-motivating-factors-mmr-vaccination-communities-low-coverage-sweden-15027.pdf

31. Tomlinson N, Redwood S. Health beliefs about preschool immunisations: an exploration of the views of Somali women resident in the UK. *Diversity and Equality in Health and Care* 2013;10:101–13.

32. Caulfield T, et al. Injecting doubt: Responding to the naturopathic anti-vaccination rhetoric. *J Law Biosci* 2017:1–21. doi:10.1093/jlb/lsx017

33. http://www.boiseweekly.com/boise/video-anti-vaccination-advocates-hold-rally-at-idaho-statehouse/Content?oid=3862113

34. Are vaccines making your child mentally ill? *The Nation* (Kenya). May 17, 2013. http://www.nation.co.ke/lifestyle/saturday/Are-vaccines-making-your-child-mentally-ill/1216-1855180-fcm005/index.html
35. Wanjohi AM. Autism in Kenya and its prevalence. 2010. KENPRO Publications. http://www.kenpro.org/papers/autism-in-kenya.htm
36. Willingham E. Court Rulings Don't Confirm Autism-Vaccine Link. *Forbes* 9 Aug 2013. https://www.forbes.com/sites/emilywillingham/2013/08/09/court-rulings-dont-confirm-autism-vaccine-link/#12babc372c88
37. Aquino F, et al. The web and public confidence in MMR vaccination in Italy. *Vaccine* 2017;35(35):4494–4498.
38. Hviid A, et al. Measles, mumps, rubella vaccination and autism. Nationwide cohort study. *Ann Intern Med* 2019;170:513–520. doi:10.7326/M18-2101
39. Manrique PD, et al. Context matters: Improving the uses of big data for forecasting civil unrest: Emerging phenomena and big data. *Proceedings of the 2013 IEEE International Conference on Intelligence and Security Informatics*, 169–172.
40. Goffman W. Generalization of epidemic theory: An application to the Transmission of Ideas. *Nature* 1964;204:225–228.
41. Daley DJ, Kendall DG. Epidemics and rumors. *Nature* 1964;204:1118.
42. Zhao L, Wang J, Chen Y, et al. SIHR rumor spreading model in social networks. *Physica A* 2012;391:2444–2453.
43. Jin F, Dougherty E, Saraf P, Cao Y, Ramakrishnan N. Epidemiological modeling of news and rumors on Twitter. *Proceedings of the 7th Workshop on Social Network Mining and Analysis* 2013;8. doi:10.1145/2501025.2501027
44. Salathé M, Khandelwal S. Assessing vaccination sentiments with online social media: Implications for infectious disease dynamics and control. *PLoS Comput Biol* 2011;7(10):e1002199.
45. Fertility regulating vaccines: Report of a meeting between women's health advocates and scientists to review the current status of the development of fertility regulating vaccines, Geneva, August 17–18, 1992.
46. http://www.physiciansforlife.org/tag/world-federation-of-doctors-who-respect-human-life/
47. Ndumbe PM, Yenshu E. Cameroon: Vaccination and politics. *Lancet* 1992;339:1222.
48. Feldman-Savelsberg P, et al. Sterilizing vaccines or the politics of the womb: Retrospective study of a rumor in Cameroon *Med Anthropol Q* June 2000;14(2):159–179.
49. Ndumbe, Yenshu. Cameroon.
50. https://apps.who.int/iris/bitstream/handle/10665/61301/WHO_HRP_WHO_93.1.pdf?sequence=1&isAllowed=y
51. Milstien J, Griffin PD, Lee JW. Damage to immunisation programmes from misinformation on contraceptive vaccines. *Reprod Health Matters* 1995;3(6):24–28.

52. Press statement by the Catholic Health Commission of Kenya, Kenya Conference of Catholic Bishops on the national tetanus vaccination campaign scheduled for 13th–19th October 2014. https://www.kccb.or.ke/home/news-2/press-statement-5/

53. Kaler A. Health interventions and the persistence of rumour: The circulation of sterility stories in African public health campaigns. *Soc Sci Med* 2009;68:1711–1719.

54. Njeru I, et al. Did the call for boycott by the Catholic bishops affect the polio vaccination coverage in Kenya in 2015? A cross-sectional study. *Pan African Med J* 2016;24:120. doi:10.11604/pamj.2016.24.120.8986

55. https://www.npr.org/sections/goatsandsoda/2015/08/09/430347033/catholic-bishops-in-kenya-call-for-a-boycott-of-polio-vaccines?t=1570982709357

56. https://www.voanews.com/africa/kenyas-catholic-bishops-call-polio-vaccine-boycott

Chapter 2

1. https://www.youtube.com/watch?v=qYI-dC9G0us

2. https://therefusers.com/how-to-spot-a-vaccine-zombie-video/

3. http://www.newindianexpress.com/states/karnataka/2017/jan/24/cannot-force-measles-rubella-re-vaccination-if-parents-do-not-agree-tanvir-sait-1563065.html

4. http://www.thedailysheeple.com/?s=vaccines

5. https://www.independent.co.uk/news/world/europe/bear-cliff-edge-200-sheep-france-spain-a7856001.html

6. http://www.sheeple.news/2017-07-30-169-dead-sheep-who-threw-themselves-over-a-cliff-perfectly-demonstrate-how-government-uses-fear-to-control-the-masses.html

7. http://www.samawomenshealth.in/memorandum-on-concerns-around-hpv-vaccines/

8. Larson HJ, et al. The India HPV vaccine suspension. *Lancet* 2010;376:572–573.

9. Sankaranarayanan R. Current status of human papillomavirus vaccination in India's cervical cancer prevention efforts. *Lancet Oncol* 2019;20:e637–44.

10. http://www.yakugai.gr.jp/topics/file/en/Joint%20Statement%202018%20for%20the%20Victims%20of%20HPV%20Vaccines.pdf

11. Kummervold P, et al. Controversial Ebola vaccine trials in Ghana: A thematic analysis of critiques and rebuttals in digital news. *BMC Public Health* 2017;17:642.

12. Freed GL, et al. Alternative vaccination schedule preferences among parents of young children. *Pediatrics* 2011;128:848.

13. Ireland N. Doctors worry as anti-vaccination messages escalate from social media misinformation to personal threats. https://www.cbc.ca/news/health/anti-vaccination-threats-against-canadian-doctors-1.5115955

14. Wong JC. Anti-vaxx "mobs": Doctors face harassment campaigns on Facebook. https://www.theguardian.com/technology/2019/feb/27/facebook-anti-vaxx-harassment-campaigns-doctors-fight-back

15. Personal communication.

16. NotSunkYet (re: wakefied). https://www.youtube.com/watch?v=cXst2V2RZR0

17. Wilson R. "I said no for a reason" Understanding factors influencing vaccination acceptance during pregnancy in Hackney, London. London School of Hygiene and Tropical Medicine, 2017, PhD dissertation, 83.

18. Pattison S. Dealing with uncertainty. *BMJ* 2001;323:840.

19. http://www.prnewswire.com/news-releases/vaccine-safety-documentary-widens-release-to-europe-despite-censorship-attempts-300409484.html

20. http://www.codacons.it/articoli/vaccini_codacons_denuncia_il_senato_e_il_presidente_grasso_290376.html

21. Le Bon G. *The crowd: A study of the popular mind.* New York: Macmillan Co., 1896.

22. https://www.homeopathy-soh.org/index.php?Itemid=101&catid=10&id=317percent3Asociety-supports-che-s-debate&option=com_content&view=article

23. Caulfield T, et al. Injecting doubt: Responding to the naturopathic anti-vaccination rhetoric. *J Law Biosci* 2017:1–21. doi:10.1093/jlb/lsx017

24. https://www.independent.co.uk/news/health/andrew-wakefield-who-is-mmr-doctor-anti-vaccine-anti-vaxxer-us-a8328326.html

25. Taylor LE, et al. Vaccines are not associated with autism: An evidence-based meta-analysis of case-control and cohort studies. *Vaccine.* 2014;32(29): 3623–3629.

26. https://www.houstonchronicle.com/news/politics/texas/article/Statewide-data-shows-Texas-anti-vaccine-movement-13089963.php

27. Wechsler J. UN Pact Scuttles Anti-Vaccine Provision. January 23, 2013. http://www.pharmexec.com/un-pact-scuttles-anti-vaccine-provision-0

Chapter 3

1. Wilson R. "I said no for a reason" Understanding factors influencing vaccination acceptance during pregnancy in Hackney, London: London School of Hygiene and Tropical Medicine, 2017, PhD dissertation, 150.

2. Karafillakis E, Larson HJ. The benefit of the doubt or doubts over benefits? A systematic literature review of perceived risks of vaccines in European populations. *Vaccine* 2017;35:4840–4850.

3. Slovic P, et al. Risk as analysis and risk as feelings: Some thoughts about affect, reason, risk, and rationality. *Risk Analysis* 2004;24(2):311–322.

4. Wilson (n1) 81.

5. Kahneman D, Tversky A. Choices, values, and frames. *Am Psychologist* 1984;39(4):341–350.

6. Daniel Kahneman biography. https://www.nobelprize.org/prizes/economic-sciences/2002/kahneman/facts/

7. Lewin K. *Principles of topological psychology.* New York: McGraw-Hill, 1936, 12.

8. Barlow WE, et al. Centers for Disease Control and Prevention Vaccine Safety Datalink Working Group. The risk of seizures after receipt of whole-cell pertussis or measles, mumps, and rubella vaccine. *N Engl J Med* 2001;345(9):656–661.

9. Vestergaard M, et al. MMR vaccination and febrile seizures: Evaluation of susceptible subgroups and long-term prognosis. *JAMA* 2004;292(3):351–357.

10. Sjøgren K. Breakthrough: Why MMR vaccine can give children febrile seizures. *ScienceNordic* November 11, 2014. http://sciencenordic.com/breakthrough-why-mmr-vaccine-can-give-children-febrile-seizures

11. Feenstra B, et al. Common variants associated with general and MMR vaccine–related febrile seizures. *Nat Genetics* 2014;46:1274–1282.

12. US Centers for Disease Control (CDC). https://www.cdc.gov/vaccines/vac-gen/side-effects.htm

13. The *Vaccine Safety Net* reviews the accuracy of various websites and creates a list of recommended sites for information on vaccine safety; see https://www.vaccinesafetynet.org/

14. Children's Hospital of Philadelphia. Vaccine safety references. https://www.chop.edu/centers-programs/vaccine-education-center/vaccine-safety-references

15. Wakefield A, et al. Retracted: Ileal-lymphoid-nodular hyperplasia, non-specific colitis, and pervasive developmental disorder in children. *Lancet* 1998;351(9103):637–641.

16. Wakefield AJ, Montgomery SM. Autism, viral infection and measles-mumps-rubella vaccination. *Israel Med Assoc J* 1999;1:183–187.

17. Coghlan A. Autism rises despite MMR ban in Japan. *New Scientist,* March 3, 2005.https://www.newscientist.com/article/dn7076-autism-rises-despite-mmr-ban-in-japan/

18. Hviid A, et al. Measles, mumps, rubella vaccination and autism: A nationwide cohort study. *Ann Intern Med* March 5, 2019. doi:10.7326/M18-2101

19. Chen W, et al. No evidence for links between autism, MMR and measles virus. *Psychol Med* 2004;34(3):543–553.

20. Smeeth L, et al. MMR vaccination and pervasive developmental disorders: A case-control study. *Lancet* 2004;364(9438):963–969.

21. Fombonne E, et al. No evidence for a new variant of measles-mumps-rubella-induced autism. *Pediatrics* 2001;108(4):E58.

22. Hornig, M, et al. Lack of association between measles virus vaccine and autism with enteropathy: A case-control study. *PLoS One* 2008;3(9):e3140.
23. DeStefano R, Shimabukuro TT. The MMR vaccine and autism. *Ann Rev Virol* 2019;6:1.1–1.16.
24. Sandin S, et al. The familial risk of autism. *JAMA*. 2014;311(17):1170–1777.
25. DA Rossignol, SJ Genius, Frye RE. Environmental toxicants and autism spectrum disorders: A systematic review. *Transl Psychiatry* 2104;4:1–23.
26. See Jamuna Prasad (1935) in Chapter 1.
27. Joint Statement of AAFP, AAP, ACIP, and the USPHS on thimerosal in childhood vaccines. June 2000. http://www.vaccinesafety.edu/AAFP-AAP-ACIP-thimerosal.htm
28. Centers for Disease Control. Understanding thimerosal, mercury, and vaccine safety. https://www.fda.gov/media/83535/download
29. Institute of Medicine (IOM), Committee on the Assessment of Studies of Health Outcomes Related to the Recommended Childhood Immunizations Schedule. *Childhood immunization schedule and safety: Stakeholder concerns, scientific evidence, and future studies.* Washington, DC: National Academies Press, 2013.
30. Taylor LE, et al. Vaccines are not associated with autism: An evidence-based meta-analysis of case-control and cohort studies. *Vaccine* 2014;32(29):3623–3629.
31. Paul Offit interview on removing thiomersal as a "precautionary measure." http://straighttalkmd.com/precautionary-principle-removing-thimerosal-vaccines-hasnt-made-safer/
32. Slovic P, et al. Risk as analysis and risk as feelings: Some thoughts about affect, reason, risk, and rationality. *Risk Analysis* 2004;24(2):311–322.
33. Dorozynski A. Suspension of hepatitis B vaccination condemned. *BMJ* 1998;317:1034.
34. Balinski MA. Hepatitis B vaccination and French society ten years after the suspension. *J Clin Virol* 2009;46:202–205.
35. Balinska MA, Léon C. Opinions et réticences face à la vaccination. *Rev Med Int* 2007;28:28–32.
36. Rabesandratana T. France most skeptical about science and vaccines, global survey finds. *Science* Jun. 19, 2019. https://www.sciencemag.org/news/2019/06/france-most-skeptical-about-science-and-vaccines-global-survey-finds
37. Wellcome Global Monitor 2018. https://wellcome.ac.uk/reports/wellcome-global-monitor/2018/chapter-5-attitudes-vaccines
38. Hanley S, et al. HPV vaccination crisis in Japan. *Lancet* 2015;385(9987):2571.
39. Japan Ministry of Health Labour and Welfare. https://www.mhlw.go.jp/topics/bcg/other/5.html (Reporting 2016 HPV vaccine uptake at 0.3%.)
40. Simms KT, Hanley SJB, Smith MA, Keane A, Canfell K. Impact of HPV vaccine hesitancy on cervical cancer in Japan: a modelling study. *Lancet Public Health* 2020;5:e223–34.

41. Global Vaccine Safety Initiative. *Report of a meeting, Santiago, Chile, October 8–9, 2018.* Geneva: World Health Organization, 2019. (WHO/MVP/EMP/SAV/2019.1)

42. https://www.sciencemag.org/news/2019/04/dengue-vaccine-fiasco-leads-criminal-charges-researcher-philippines

43. Larson HJ, Hartigan-Go K, de Figueiredo A. Vaccine confidence plummets in the Philippines following dengue vaccine scare: Why it matters to pandemic preparedness. *Hum Vaccines Immunotherapeut* 2018. doi:10.1080/21645515.2018.1522468

44. The first national "risk communication" conference took place in January 1986, in Washington, DC. The "National Conference on Risk Communication," was sponsored jointly by the Environmental Protection Agency, the National Science Foundation, and the Conservation Foundation" (Sandmann, 2009 Berreth Lecture).

45. Sandman P. *Hazards vs. outrage: Responding to community outrage,* 1993. http://psandman.com/media/RespondingtoCommunityOutrage.pdf

46. Fischoff B. Risk perception and communication unplugged: Twenty years of process. *Risk Analysis* 1995;15(2):137–144.

47. Pidgeon, N., Kasperson, R., & Slovic, P. (eds.). *The Social Amplification of Risk.* Cambridge: Cambridge University Press, 2003.

Chapter 4

1. Williamson S. One hundred years ago. Anti-Vaccination Leagues. *Arch Dis Child* 1984;59:1195–1196.

2. TEA/AECOM. 2014 Theme index and museum index: The global attractions attendance report. http://www.teaconnect.org/images/files/TEA_103_49736_150603.pdf Accessed June 12, 2017.

3. https://leginfo.legislature.ca.gov/faces/billNavClient.xhtml?bill_id=201520160SB277

4. https://www.sott.net/article/297819-Medical-tyranny-California-Vaccine-SB277-Bill-passes-Health-Committee

5. http://www.nvic.org/nvic-vaccine-news/july-2015/california-sb277-enacted-end-medical-tryanny.aspx

6. California Department of Public Health, Immunization Branch. 2017–2018 kindergarten immunization assessment—executive summary. https:// www.cdph.ca.gov/ Programs/ CID/ DCDC/ CDPHpercent20Documentpercent20Library/Immunization/ 2017- 2018KindergartenSummaryReport. pdf

7. Mohanty S, Buttenheim AM, Joyce CM, et al. Experiences with medical exemptions after a change in vaccine exemption policy in California. *Pediatrics* 2018;142(5):e20181051.

8. https://www.kqed.org/news/11742525/california-lawmakers-consider-crackdown-on-fake-medical-exemptions-for-vaccines

9. https://leginfo.legislature.ca.gov/faces/billTextClient.xhtml?bill_id=201920200SB276

10. https://www.nytimes.com/2019/04/26/us/measles-outbreak-los-angeles-quarantine.html

11. Esch M. Unvaccinated children banned from public spaces in N.Y. county. March 27, 2019. https://globalnews.ca/news/5101034/new-york-vaccination-ban/

12. https://www.cnbc.com/2019/04/19/judge-upholds-new-york-citys-mandatory-measles-vaccination-order.html

13. https://www.buzzfeednews.com/article/claudiakoerner/anti-vaccine-peach-measles-new-york-propaganda-outbreak

14. Tabachnick T. Anon Anonymous anti-vaxxers push propaganda on local Orthodox community. January 31, 2018. https://jewishchronicle.timesofisrael.com/anonymous-anti-vaxxers-push-propaganda-on-local-orthodox-community/

15. http://nymag.com/intelligencer/2019/09/california-vaccination-law-draws-protests-no-segregation.html

16. https://www.theroot.com/we-shall-over-whomst-white-anti-vaxxers-colonize-civil-1838256562

17. DiResta R. Of virality and viruses: The anti-vaccine movement and social media. NAPSNet Special Reports. November 8, 2018. https://nautilus.org/napsnet/napsnet-special-reports/of-virality-and-viruses-the-anti-vaccine-movement-and-socialmedia/

18. BBC Radio 4, September 30, 2019.

19. https://elpais.com/elpais/2015/06/05/inenglish/1433512717_575817.html

20. http://www.euro.who.int/en/media-centre/sections/press-releases/2018/europe-observes-a-4-fold-increase-in-measles-cases-in-2017-compared-to-previous-year

21. https://www.msuilr.org/msuilr-legalforum-blogs/2017/11/30/mandatory-vaccination-in-in-france

22. Ward J, et al. Why France is making eight new vaccines mandatory. *Vaccine* 2018;36:1801–1803.

23. Extension of French vaccination mandates: From the recommendation of the Steering Committee of the Citizen Consultation on Vaccination to the law. https://www.eurosurveillance.org/content/10.2807/1560-7917.ES.2018.23.17.18-00048

24. https://www.politico.eu/article/vaccine-debate-gives-italian-election-campaign-a-shot-in-the-arm/

25. http://www.ansa.it/english/news/2018/06/22/salvini-says-having-10-obligatory-vaccines-useless-3_8bcb2b7d-2217-444f-ac30-1914a82a89fe.html

26. https://www.independent.co.uk/news/health/italian-health-chief-quits-anti-vaxx-measles-populist-walter-ricciardi-a8713126.html?utm_term=Autofeed&utm_medium=Social&utm_source=Twitter#Echobox=1546710065

27. Giuffrida A. Sacking of Italy's health experts raises political interference concerns. *The Guardian.* December 4, 2018. https://www.theguardian.com/world/2018/dec/04/politically-motivated-italys-m5s-sacks-peak-board-of-health-experts

28. https://www.independent.co.uk/news/health/italian-health-chief-quits-anti-vaxx-measles-populist-walter-ricciardi-a8713126.html?utm_term=Autofeed&utm_medium=Social&utm_source=Twitter#Echobox=1546710065

29. https://ilglobo.com.au/news/41331/italys-health-minister-sacks-entire-board-of-experts/

30. Esch. Sacking of Italy's health experts.

31. 1998 Beppe Grillo "Soft Apocalypse" performance on vaccines. https://www.youtube.com/watch?v=xemA2zX7y7w

32. Friedman U. What is a Populist? *The Atlantic.* February 27, 2017. https://www.theatlantic.com/international/archive/2017/02/what-is-populist-trump/516525/

33. Kennedy J. Populist politics and vaccine hesitancy in Western Europe: An analysis of national-level data. *Eur J Pub Health* 2019;29(3):512–516.

34. Lasco G, Curato N. Medical populism. *Soc Sci Med* 2019;221:1–8.

35. Friedman. What is a Populist?

36. Karnad R. It's not what Modi is tweeting—It's what he is reading. *The Wire.* September 2, 2017. https://thewire.in/107145/narendra-modi-twitter-trolls/

37. https://www.euronews.com/2018/06/02/thousands-of-people-in-warsaw-protested-against-compulsory-vaccinations

38. Zuk P, et al. The anti-vaccine movement in Poland: The socio-cultural conditions of the opposition to vaccination and threats to public health. *Vaccine* 2019;37:1491–1494.

39. Bielecki K, et al. Low uptake of nasal influenza vaccine in Polish and other ethnic minority children in Edinburgh, Scotland. *Vaccine* 2019 Jan 29;37(5):693–697. doi:10.1016/j.vaccine.2018.11.029. Epub November 16, 2018.

40. Pollock KG, et al. Evidence of decreased HPV vaccine acceptance in Polish communities within Scotland. *Vaccine* 2019 Jan 29;37(5):690–692. doi:10.1016/j.vaccine.2018.10.097

41. Porter D, Porter R. The politics of prevention: Antivaccinationism and public health in nineteenth century England. *Med Hist* 1988;32:231–252.

42. Swales JD. The Leicester anti-vaccination movement. *Lancet* 1992; 340(8826):1019–1021.

43. Mill JS. *On liberty*. London: Penguin Books (1974 edition), 67.
44. *Leicester Mercury*. June 10, 1884. (Referenced in Wiliamson S. One hundred years ago Anti-Vaccination Leagues. *Arch Dis Child* 1984;59:1195–1196.
45. Swales JD,1020.
46. Novak S. The long history of America's anti-vaccination movement. December 2018. http://discovermagazine.com/2018/dec/fostering-fear

Chapter 5

1. https://www.nytimes.com/2018/08/13/science/wildfires-physics.html
2. 2009 Victorian Royal Commission bushfires final report. July 2010. http://royalcommission.vic.gov.au/finaldocuments/summary/PF/VBRC_Summary_PF.pdf
3. Attiwill P, Binkley D. Exploring the mega-fire reality: A "forest ecology and management" conference. *Forest Ecology Management* 2013;294:1–3.
4. Arango T, Medina J. California fire now the largest in state history: "People are on edge." https://www.nytimes.com/2018/08/07/us/california-fires-mendocino.html?module=inline
5. https://www.seattletimes.com/seattle-news/inslee-declares-wildfire-state-of-emergency-in-washington/
6. Robbins J. Fierce and unpredictable: How wildfires became infernos. https://www.nytimes.com/2018/08/13/science/wildfires-physics.html
7. Yeung J. Australia's deadly wildfires are showing no signs of stopping. Here's what you need to know https://edition.cnn.com/2020/01/01/australia/australia-fires-explainer-intl-hnk-scli/index.html
8. Kay J. The enduring certainty of radical uncertainty. https://www.ft.com/content/ec5520c4-fb23-11e5-8f41-df5bda8beb40
9. Mishra P. *Age of anger: A history of the present*. London: Penguin Books, 2017.
10. https://www.washingtonpost.com/national/health-science/it-will-take-off-like-a-wildfire-the-unique-dangers-of-the-washington-state-measles-outbreak/2019/02/06/cfd5088a-28fa-11e9-b011-d8500644dc98_story.html?utm_term=.b9bc09f628aa
11. https://www.clark.wa.gov/public-health/faq/what-are-immunization-rates-children-clark-county
12. http://www.euro.who.int/en/media-centre/sections/press-releases/2019/measles-in-europe-record-number-of-both-sick-and-immunized
13. https://www.physiciansweekly.com/alarming-upsurge-in-measles/
14. World Economic Forum. *Global Risks 2013*. http://www3.weforum.org/docs/WEF_GlobalRisks_Report_2013.pdf
15. Johnson NF, et al. Hidden resilience and adaptive dynamics of the global on-line hate ecology. *Nature* 2019; 573, 261–265.

16. https://scroll.in/pulse/830129/rumours-about-measles-rubella-vaccine-hit-coverage

17. https://timesofindia.indiatimes.com/city/meerut/madrassas-in-west-up-say-no-to-measles-rubella-vaccination/articleshow/67184011.cms

18. https://www.msn.com/en-in/news/jobs-education/mumbai-measles-rubella-vaccination-blocked-as-fake-news-of-infertility-spreads-on-social-media/vp-BBSgxgr

19. https://www.pri.org/stories/2019-04-24/india-whatsapp-weapon-antisocial-hatred

20. https://timesofindia.indiatimes.com/india/Congress-vs-BJP-The-curious-case-of-trolls-and-politics/articleshow/23970818.cms?utm_source=contentofinterest&utm_medium=text&utm_campaign=cppst

21. Peckham R, ed. *Empires of panic.* Hong Kong: Hong Kong University Press, 2015, 5.

22. Garrett L. The real reason to panic about China's plague outbreak. *Foreign Affairs.* November 16, 2019.| https://foreignpolicy.com/2019/11/16/china-bubonic-plague-outbreak-pandemic/

23. Deb A, Donohue S, Glaisyer T. *Is social media a threat to democracy?* ebook: Omidyar Group, 2017. https://www.com/wp-content/uploads/2017/10/Social-Media-and-Democracy-October-5-2017.pdf

24. https://news.harvard.edu/gazette/story/2018/10/martin-rees-brings-on-the-future-prospects-for-humanity-to-harvard/

25. https://www.npr.org/sections/thetwo-way/2018/01/22/579732762/facebook-says-social-media-can-be-negative-for-democracy

26. Diamond L, Plattner MF, eds. *Liberation Technology: Social Media and the Struggle for Democracy.* Baltimore: The Johns Hopkins University Press, 2012.

27. World Economic Forum, 28.

28. Farmer B. Fake vaccine video goes viral in Pakistan putting the global drive to eradicate polio at risk at the 11th hour. https://www.telegraph.co.uk/global-health/science-and-disease/fake-vaccine-video-goes-viral-pakistan-putting-global-drive/

29. https://www.youtube.com/watch?v=wKqsR4C3T84

30. https://www.telegraph.co.uk/news/2018/07/07/fake-vaccine-video-goes-viral-pakistan-putting-global-drive/

31. https://www.france24.com/en/20190503-pakistan-demands-facebook-remove-polio-vaccine-misinformation

32. https://www.japantimes.co.jp/news/2019/05/03/asia-pacific/science-health-asia-pacific/monstrous-rumors-stoke-hostility-pakistans-anti-polio-drive/#.XM4Mh0hKjD4

33. Yinka-Ogunleye A, Aruna O, Ogoina D, et al. Reemergence of Human Monkeypox in Nigeria, 2017. *Emerging Infectious Diseases.* 2018;24(6): 1149–1151.

34. The monkey pox vaccine hoax. http://thepointernewsonline.com/?p=56710
35. https://www.express.co.uk/news/world/878464/the-plague-madagascar-2017-doctor-black-death-school-stampede-vaccine-pnuemonic
36. https://www.who.int/csr/don/27-november-2017-plague-madagascar/en/
37. https://madagascar-tribune.com/Rumeur-de-vaccination-forcee-et,23427.html
38. Kirby W. Black death stampede: Panic in Madagascar amid plague vaccination fury. *Express*. https://www.express.co.uk/news/world/878464/the-plague-madagascar-2017-doctor-black-death-school-stampede-vaccine-pnuemonic
39. https://www.telegraphindia.com/states/odisha/girl-s-body-exhumed-for-probe/cid/1407826
40. https://www.reuters.com/article/us-sanofi-dengue-philippines/philippines-exhumes-bodies-of-two-children-in-dengue-vaccine-probe-idUSKBN1F01AY
41. https://schiff.house.gov/news/press-releases/schiff-sends-letter-to-google-facebook-regarding-anti-vaccine-misinformation
42. https://www.adweek.com/digital/ama-letter-implores-tech-companies-to-do-more-about-vaccine-misinformation/
43. Smyth C. Anti-vaccine posts could be banned from social media. *The Times* (UK). March 27, 2019.
44. https://motherboard.vice.com/en_us/article/xwk9zd/how-facebook-content-moderation-works
45. https://www.nbcnews.com/tech/social-media/now-available-more-200-000-deleted-russian-troll-tweets-n844731
46. https://www.theguardian.com/technology/2018/jul/19/facebook-fake-news-violence-moderation-plan
47. Wolchover N. The Physicist Modeling ISIS and the Alt-Right. The Atlantic August 28, 2017 *https://www.theatlantic.com/science/archive/2017/08/the-physicist-modeling-isis-and-the-alt-right/537699/*
48. UN Human Rights Council. 38th Session. June–July 2018.[A/HRC/38/35]Report of the Special Rapporteur on the promotion and protection of the right to freedom of opinion and expression. https://freedex.org/wp-content/blogs.dir/2015/files/2018/05/G1809672.pdf
49. McLuhan M. *Understanding media: The extensions of man.* Cambridge, MA: MIT Press, 1964.
50. https://www.totallydublin.ie/film/technologic-interview-godfrey-reggio/

Chapter 6

1. See William McDougall (1920) in Introduction.
2. Carlos Guevara M. Class action lawsuit against HPV vaccine filed in Colombia. Medscape. August 7, 2017. http://www.medscape.com/viewarticle/883873

3. Larson HJ. Global girl gang. *Lancet* 2018;391:527–528.

4. Sartori A. "HPV introduction in Brazilian schools: lessons learnt for dengue vaccine introduction" Presentation at "Pre-vaccination screening for the use of dengue vaccines widifferential performance dependent on serostatus: rapid dinostic tests and implementation strategies" meeting aMerieux Foundation, Annecy. January 14, 2019. https://www.gdac-dengue.org/wp-content/uploads/2019/02/dengue-pre-vaccination-screening-based-on-serostatus-2019-report.pdf

5. Chapman S, MacKenzie R. Fainting schoolgirls wipe $A1bn off market value of Gardasil producer. *BMJ* 2007;334:1195

6. https://www.youtube.com/watch?v=BGjn1ZOnRiY#action=share

7. Suzuki S, Hosono A. No association between HPV vaccine and reported post-vaccination symptoms in Japanese young women: Results of the Nagoya study. *Papillomavirus Res.* 2018;5:96–103.

8. Konno R, et al. Effectiveness of HPV vaccination against high grade cervical lesions in Japan. *Vaccine* 2018;36:7913–7915.

9. Larson HJ, Wilson R, Hanley S et al. Tracking the global spread of vaccine sentiments: The global response to Japan's suspension of its HPV vaccine recommendation. *Hum Vaccines Immunotherapeut* 2014;10(9): 2543–2550.

10. https://www.belfasttelegraph.co.uk/life/health/a-belfastmans-quest-to-find-out-if-a-simple-vitamin-pill-can-beat-some-of-our-cruellest-illnesses-34319329.html

11. file:///C:/Users/eidehlar/Downloads/Proposal%20for%20HPV%20demo%20application%202017%20-%20Armenia.pdf

12. Berlier M, et al. Communication challenges during the development and introduction of a new meningococcal vaccine in Africa. *CID* 2015;61(Suppl 5):S451.

13. Yang TU. Psychogenic illness following vaccination: Exploratory study of mass vaccination against pandemic influenza A (H1N1) in 2009 in South Korea. *Clin Exp Vaccine Res* 2017;6:31–37.

14. http://www.who.int/vaccine_safety/committee/topics/global_AEFI_monitoring/Dec_2015/en/

15. Kharabsheh S, et al. Mass psychogenic illness following tetanus-diphtheria toxoid vaccination in Jordan. *Bull WHO* 2001;79:764–770.

16. Yasamy MT, et al. Post vaccination mass psychogenic illness in an Iranian rural school. *Eastern Mediterranean Health Journal* 1999;5(4):710–716.

17. Bartholomew RE, Wessely S. Protean nature of mass sociogenic illness: From possessed nuns to chemical and biological terrorism fears. *Br J Psychiatry* 2002 Apr;180:300–306.

18. Nemery B, et al. The Coca-Cola incident in Belgium, June 1999. *Food Chem Toxicol* 2002;40:1657–1667.

19. Taylor M. Cultural variance as a challenge to global public relations: A case study of the Coca-Cola scare in Europe. *Public Relations Rev* 2000;26(3):277–293.
20. http://www.nytimes.com/2012/03/11/magazine/teenage-girls-twitching-le-roy.html?_r=1
21. Bartholomew RE, Wessely S, Rubin JG. Mass psychogenic illness and the social network: Is it changing the pattern of outbreaks? *J R Soc Med* 2012;105:509–512.
22. Bates D. Facebook to blame for the panic surrounding mysterious Tourettes-like illness spreading in rural New York town. *DailyMail* (UK). February 5, 2012. https://www.dailymail.co.uk/news/article-2096813/Could-infection-mysterious-Tourettes-like-syndrome-affecting-teenagers.html
23. Wessely S. Mass hysteria: Two syndromes?*Psychol Med* 1987;17:109–20.
24. Bartholomew RE. Mass psychogenic illness and the social network.
25. Kramer ADI, Guillory JE, Hancock JT. Experimental evidence of massive-scale emotional contagion through social networks. *PNAS* 2014;111(29):10779.
26. Loharikar A, et al. Anxiety-related adverse events following immunization (AEFI): A systematic review of published clusters of illness. *Vaccine* 2017. https://www.ncbi.nlm.nih.gov/pubmed/29198916
27. World Health Organization (WHO). *Immunization stress-related response. A manual for program managers and health professionals to prevent, identify and respond to stressrelated responses following immunization.* Geneva: World Health Organization; 2019. https://www.who.int/publications-detail/978-92-4-151594-8

Chapter 7

1. *Calpol* is the brand name for a UK product used to treat infant fevers and colds.
2. https://www.npr.org/sections/health-shots/2011/11/07/142098710/what-not-to-buy-online-lollipops-laced-with-chickenpox
3. https://www.theglobeandmail.com/life/the-hot-button/how-many-licks-does-it-take-to-get-chicken-pox-parents-trade-vaccines-for-lollipops/article619035/
4. Harford T. The pseudoscience of Blue Monday hits trust. *Financial Times,* January 26, 2019.
5. Sabahelzain MM, et al. Towards a further understanding of measles vaccine hesitancy in Khartoum state, Sudan: A qualitative study. *PLoS One* 2019;14(6):e0213882.
6. http://www.immunize.org/talking-about-vaccines/porcine.pdf
7. Latiff R. Some Malaysians' rejection of vaccines fans fears of disease surge. July 6, 2016. Reuters. https://www.reuters.com/article/malaysia-vaccine-idUSL4N19R1KF

8. https://www.thenewsminute.com/article/after-diphtheria-anti-vaccination-groups-oppose-measles-rubella-shot-kerala-govt-steps-69574

9. https://www.buzzfeed.com/elfyscott/vaccines-are-not-halal-and-that-can-be-a-big-problem-for

10. https://www.abc.net.au/news/2018-01-15/islamic-anti-vaxxers-undermining-diphtheria-vaccination-campaign/9325852

11. Hussain A, et al. The anti-vaccination movement: A regression in modern medicine. *Cureus* 2018;10(7):e2919. doi:10.7759/cureus.2919

12. Walsh D. Polio cases jump in Pakistan as clerics declare vaccination an American plot. *The Guardian.* https://www.theguardian.com/world/2007/feb/15/pakistan.topstories3

13. Kennedy J, et al. Islamist insurgency and the war against polio: A cross-national analysis of the political determinants of polio. *Globalization Health* 2015;11:40.

14. Ledwith M. Tragic death of the Afghan girl who just wanted to change her country: Student shot dead as she helped in fight against polio. *Daily Mail* December 6, 2012. https://www.dailymail.co.uk/news/article-2244133/Afghan-girl-Anisa-worked-polio-volunteer-shot-dead-suspected-Taliban-attack.html

15. http://www.diseasedaily.org/diseasedaily/article/least-nine-polio-workers-killed-nigeria-21113

16. Iganatius D. A CIA gambit in Pakistan threatens a global vaccination program. *Washington Post.* May 29, 2012. https://www.washingtonpost.com/opinions/a-cia-gambit-in-pakistan-threatens-a-global-vaccination-program/2012/05/29/gJQAW6W1zU_story.html?noredirect=on&utm_term=.feef547a7d6b

17. http://www.virology.ws/2013/01/08/deans-write-to-obama-about-cia-vaccine-scheme-in-pakistan/

18. McKenna M. Polio returns to Nigeria for the first time in years. *National Geographic.* August 12, 2016. https://news.nationalgeographic.com/2016/08/new-polio-cases-in-nigeria-africa-vaccinations/

19. https://www.scidev.net/south-asia/conflict/news/taliban-kill-15-people-attack-polio-centre.html

20. https://www.aljazeera.com/news/2019/04/gunmen-kill-polio-vaccinator-southwestern-pakistan-190425105934848.html

21. http://www.polioeradication.org/Portals/0/Document/Aboutus/Governance/IMB/7IMBMeeting/7IMB_Report_EN.pd

22. Akil L, Ahmad HA. The recent outbreaks and re-emergence of poliovirus in war and conflict-affected areas. *J Infect Dis* 2016;49:40–46.

23. McGirk T. How the bin Laden raid put vaccinators under the gun in Pakistan. https://news.nationalgeographic.com/2015/02/150225-polio-pakistan-vaccination-virus-health/

Chapter 8

1. The 1918 influenza pandemic was also an H1N1 strain of the virus, which heightened public health concerns when it returned in 2009.
2. Theuns-De Boer G. Bubonic plague in Bombay, 1896–1914. *IIAS Newsletter.* https://iias.asia/iiasn/25/regions/25SA1.html
3. Barrett R, Brown PJ. Stigma in the time of influenza: Social and institutional responses to pandemic emergencies. *J Infect Dis* 2008 Feb 15;197(Suppl 1):S34-S7.
4. Peckham R. *Empires of panic: Epidemics and colonial anxieties.* Hong Kong: Hong Kong University Press, 2015, 18.
5. Leeder S. Epidemiology in an age of anger and complaint. *Intl J Epidemiol* 2017;46(1):1.
6. Sturcke J, Bowcott O. Drug companies face European inquiry over swine flu vaccine stockpiles. *The Guardian.* January 11, 2010. http://www.theguardian.com/world/2010/jan/11/swine-flu-h1n1-vaccine-europe
7. Cohen D, Carter P. WHO and the pandemic flu conspiracies. *BMJ* 2010;340:c2912.
8. http://www1.rfi.fr/actuen/articles/121/article_6381.asp; Watel P et al. Dramatic change in public attitudes towards vaccination during the 2009 influenza A(H1N1) pandemic in France. *Euro Surveill* 2013;18(44):20623. hlps://doi.org/10.2807/1560-7917.ES2013.18.44.20623 PMID: 24176658
9. Ofri D. The emotional epidemiology of H1N1 influenza vaccination. *NEJM* 2009;361;27.
10. Black S, Ruppuoli R. A crisis of public confidence in vaccines. *SciTransMed* 2010 Dec 8;2(61):61mr1.
11. https://www.cdc.gov/flu/about/burden/estimates.htm#table1
12. https://edition.cnn.com/2017/04/02/health/unseen-enemy-deadly-influenza-epidemic-gwen-zwanziger/index.html
13. https://www.theverge.com/2019/3/5/18251807/senate-anti-vax-vaccines-congressional-hearing-ethan-lindenberger-ohio-teen
14. https://www.reddit.com/r/IAmA/comments/apxlfk/im_ethan_an_18_year_old_who_made_national/
15. Davies, P., Chapman, S., Leask, J. Anitvaccination activists on the world wide web. *Archives of Disease in Childhood* 2002;87(1):22–25.
16. Wolfe RM, Sharp LK. Antivaccinationists past and present. *BMJ* 2002; 325:430–432.
17. https://www.nobelprize.org/prizes/peace/1964/king/26142-martin-luther-king-jr-acceptance-speech-1964/
18. Oldstone MBA. *Viruses, plagues and history.* New York: Oxford University Press, 2000.
19. Chen RT Evaluation of vaccine safety after the events of 11 September 2001: role of cohort and case-control studies. *Vaccine* 2004;22:2047–2053.

INDEX

Page numbers followed by n indicate endnotes.

For the benefit of digital users, indexed terms that span two pages (e.g., 52–53) may, on occasion, appear on only one of those pages.